THE ULTIMATE KETOGENIC FITNESS BOOK

A Complete Guide to Optimizing Keto for a Better Quality of Life

Written by: Bronson Dant CCFT, CPT

Disclaimer:

This book is not intended as a substitute for the medical advice of physicians. The reader should consult a physician in matters relating to his/her health and particularly with respect to any symptoms that may require diagnosis or medical attention.

This book details the author's personal experiences with and opinions about nutrition and fitness. The author is not a [or your] healthcare provider.

The statements made about products and services have not been evaluated by the U.S. Food and Drug Administration. They are not intended to diagnose, treat, cure, or prevent any condition or disease. Please consult with your own physician or healthcare specialist regarding the suggestions and recommendations made in this book.

Except as specifically stated in this book, the author, nor any authors, contributors, or other representatives will be liable for damages arising out of or in connection with the use of this book. This is a comprehensive limitation of liability that applies to all damages of any kind, including (without limitation) compensatory; direct, indirect or consequential damages; loss of data, income or profit; loss of or damage to property and claims of third parties.

You understand that this book is not intended as a substitute for consultation with a licensed healthcare practitioner, such as your physician. Before you begin any healthcare program, or change your lifestyle in any way, you will consult your physician or another licensed healthcare practitioner to ensure that you are in good health and that the examples contained in this book will not harm you.

This book provides content related to physical and/or mental health issues. As such, use of this book implies your acceptance of this disclaimer.

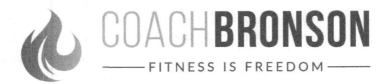

COACH**BRONSON**

——— FITNESS IS FREEDOM ———

When you're finished reading this book, you will be looking for ways to make some changes and start moving in the right direction. Lucky for you, I've created programs to help you get started!

My F2 Method Programs are the only programs that combine all the concepts from this book and my years of practical, hands-on experience into one solution. No matter where you are, there's a way for you to get started.

Find out which program will work best for you! Take the quiz here: https://coachbronson.com/quiz/

SCAN ME

Table of Contents

Foreword

Currently, over 37 million Americans have been diagnosed with diabetes, and another 96 million have pre-diabetes. Over 181 million U.S. citizens have been diagnosed as overweight, 104 million with obesity, and 22 million with severe obesity. Keep in mind, these numbers represent the number of souls who have seen a doctor and have been diagnosed; there are many millions of others who suffer with these afflictions, who have not yet been diagnosed. The way of eating that leads to these dangerous conditions also leads to many other metabolic dysfunctions, one of which is mitochondrial dysfunction. This dysfunction becomes meaningful when one of these people is given the standard advice by their healthcare provider. We've all heard it before, "you need to eat less and move more".

The "move more" half of this well-intentioned, but worthless advice, means start exercising, and here is where many run into trouble. For the vast majority of folks suffering from chronic metabolic disease, mitochondrial number and quality have degraded to such a point that the only exercise they are capable of is shuffling the quadrangle from the couch to the kitchen to the bathroom to the bed. Telling someone with such crippled biochemistry to start a daily vigorous exercise program is both unhelpful and definitionally judgmental of their ability and their motivation. This person is no more able to exercise vigorously than a monkey is to discover a law of physics. There is a vital first step needed to revive their mitochondrial numbers and rejuvenate mitochondrial function before expecting them to have enough energy to do more than the most basic activities of daily living.

When someone suffering from such metabolic disease adopts a Proper Human Diet – a low-carbohydrate, nutrient-dense, ancestrally-appropriate diet full of healthy fats and healthy proteins – many steps in their metabolic function begin to improve. This can be seen in the return of their blood glucose and insulin levels towards the normal range, the falling of their blood pressure and triglycerides back towards normal, an increase in lean body mass percentage, and a steady lowering of their body-fat percentage. And, to many a patient's surprise, their levels of energy and motivation start to increase. After some weeks or months of eating such a diet daily (after giving their mitochondria time to heal and multiply), they very naturally have the idea that today would be a good day to get in a little exercise.

The low-carb community is, by definition, a paradigm-shifting lot; they are very good at thinking about problems from different angles than the standard one. They tend to question everything and pick at standard dogma and recommendations like the worn and tattered fibers that they are. Therefore, in this community, we see an increasingly active debate about whether the goal should be to decrease body fat or to increase lean mass. There is much research on this subject, and most of it can be interpreted either way. My answer to this question is, I don't really care, the patient wins either way! Correcting a bad diet is the fundamental change that must occur to make any of these things happen, and to give this person the improved mitochondrial numbers and functionality required to have the surplus of energy needed to even consider participating in some kind of exercise program. Thankfully, many thousands of people all over the world are rediscovering a Proper Human Diet, healing their metabolisms, and rebuilding their intracellular energy plants to the point where today is that day when it occurs to them that being more active might be great fun. But now, they are faced with the fact that after decades of being completely sedentary, they don't really know how to exercise safely, or even really where to start. Here, for this population, my good friend Bronson has stepped in to save the day.

Rediscovering how to live an exercise-filled proper human life is something most of us knew intuitively as children, we just went outside and played. But, for the person over forty, sedentary for decades, it becomes very important to know *how* to start, at what intensity to start, and how to increase this intensity. I've seen many hundreds of such folks in my practice who, due to the sheer enjoyment of the exercise they were now able to do, overdid it either in the degree of resistance, or in excessive repetition, and wound up with an injury to a joint, tendon, or muscle. With proper instruction about how to begin from where you currently are, how to establish rational goals, and how to increase the intensity of exercise at the proper rate so as not to lead to injury, this book gives very clear and simple instructions on how to "go outside and play" regardless of your age, or the current depth of your sedentary spiral.

Increasing your muscle mass, bone strength, agility, and proprioception is vital if your goal is to neither look nor act your age. Bronson is just the person to show you the way. This book is a vital resource for those of us who have returned to eating like a human, and are now ready to start moving and playing like one.

Ken D Berry, MD
Author: Lies My Doctor Told Me

About the Author

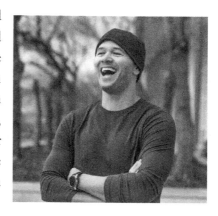

Bronson Dant has coached and trained people in health and fitness for over ten years. He started CrossFit around his 40th birthday and quickly fell in love with the variety, community, coaching, and results. It didn't take long for him to realize that learning more about fitness and becoming a coach was his life's next path.

Bronson opened a CrossFit gym in 2014. As a gym owner, helping people develop their health and fitness, Bronson designed several programs to improve his client's quality of life and physical freedom consistently and sustainably.

In 2018 Bronson discovered that following a carnivore lifestyle was the secret to the optimization of his metabolic health and performance. Since then, he has designed specific methods to use both nutrition and fitness to radically improve the lives of people all over the world.

Certifications and Training:

- CrossFit Certified Trainer (CCFT)
- Certified Personal Trainer (NASM)
- USA Powerlifting Coach (USAPL)
- USA Weightlifting Coach (USAW)
- Certified Strength and Conditioning Coach

- Functional Movement Screen
- Professional Training in LCHF/Ketogenic Nutrition & Treatment

Bronson is a frequent guest and subject matter expert on health and fitness podcasts and YouTube channels. He is also a prolific speaker and presenter at health and fitness events all over the US.

Introduction

The book you are about to read is very important. It's a collection of knowledge from years of training, lessons learned, and experiences that I've had as a Personal Trainer, CrossFit Coach, Gym Owner, and Online Nutrition and Fitness Coach.

More specifically, it's all stuff that I had to learn to help myself live the life that I wanted to live and then help others do the same.

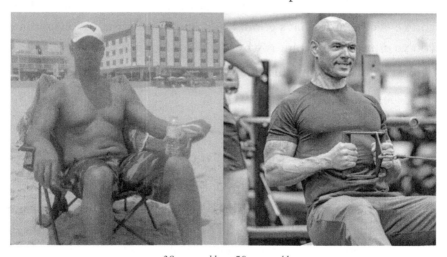

38 years old vs. 50 years old

I was just like you probably are in some way. I was out of shape. I was discouraged. I had little desire to change. I didn't know how, even if I wanted to.

When I started, I made some progress and saw some changes, but I could never seem to get to the level of health, physical performance, confidence, and happiness I was looking for. It took one thing, one mental adjustment, to make all the difference.

I forgot what I thought I knew, and I realized that what I was doing wasn't working, and I tried something new.

At the time, CrossFit was considered crazy and unsafe, but I tried it, and I loved it. It made a huge difference in my understanding of what fitness was really about. It gave me a passion and a purpose.

How my body performed and healed took a giant leap forward when I started focusing on eating the most nutrient-dense foods I could and stopped eating things that were holding my health in check. Again, I heard that I was being crazy and unsafe, but I did it anyway. I'm glad I did.

After years of living my best life and helping hundreds of other people have the same experience, here I am.

There are things in this book that will be different from anything you've ever heard. That's good. Everything you know and everything you've done to this point is why you're looking for help.

It's time for something new.

Coach Bronson

"Fitness is Freedom and Freedom is Your Choice"

P.S. I want what's best for you. This book will give you information and make you think. It's not a feel-good read. Excuses and soft truth never helped anyone make a major change. If making a change is why you're here, keep reading!

My Mom

I want to introduce you to my mom, Claire. My mom has been my client for almost 10 years.

My mom has been with me through much of the development of my methods. She's been a guinea pig for some of them. Her story is pretty amazing.

I asked her to share her story because I want you to know that this book is for you. Everything in this book is possible. I know because I've watched my mom do it.

She is the best example I have of how the information you are about to read can change your life.

My Fitness Journey, Claire Dant, Age 68

At the end of 2014, as I approached the age of 61, I was very aware that without some type of intervention, my body would continue the decline that I had experienced in the previous decade. I had been losing approximately 2.5% of bone density annually and had finally arrived at the official diagnosis of osteoporosis! This was very concerning to me, and I knew that the only way to arrest this decline was to begin some serious weight-bearing exercise.

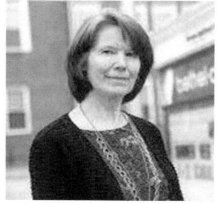

Enter CrossFit PCR, now Ellicott City Health and Fitness (ECHF). In January 2015, I began participating in CrossFit training with the hope of stemming the decline in bone density. Never having been athletic or attended a gym of any kind, this was very intimidating to me. Bronson provided personal training for a month before I joined the CrossFit classes.

I was glad to see that everything was scalable to my needs and current level of ability. It was also quite amazing to experience the camaraderie that existed with the athletes in the classes. (At that time, it was impossible to consider *myself* an athlete.) No one ever indicated that they were disappointed in what I could do, and everyone was always encouraging and supportive. My goal was to "show up and do what the coaches tell me to do."

Over the years, I continued to "do CrossFit" and saw measurable progress in my fitness level. As a person who needs results to keep me motivated, I was happy that they were so clear.

First, the progression of my osteoporosis was halted! A bone density scan after 2.5 years of CrossFit training resulted in NO additional loss of bone mass! And this was without additional bone density drugs or even calcium. I began taking a new form of calcium-based on an organic source (AlgaeCal) in January 2018. As they "guarantee" an INCREASE in bone mass in one year, I was anxious to have another scan, but my doctor wouldn't order one for another year, so I kept doing CrossFit and taking AlgaeCal and waited.

In February 2020, another bone density scan was conducted, and I had gained from 13 % - 33% bone mass at various sites. I no longer had osteoporosis in my spine – it was normal!

Because at ECHF, we were encouraged to keep track of our performances, I also have measurable results regarding my performance progress. I saw gains in strength, speed, and ability to do movements that I was not able to perform in the beginning. For example, from barbell lifts with just the 15-lb. training bar, I was able to push press

60 lbs. overhead. I could deadlift 155 pounds and bench press 65 lbs. My front squat is 75 lbs. and my back squat is 95 lbs.

I can now finish workouts within the time cap more frequently and can heft a 10-lb. medicine ball to the 9-ft. target on the wall. When I began CrossFit, I couldn't really jump; now, I can jump onto a 20-inch box. I can jump rope, row, run, and bike distances and times I would never have thought possible!

Another way I have seen progress is through my participation in the CrossFit Open for the last several years. My performance of the Open workouts in comparison to other women in my age group and division went from the bottom third the first year to the top third last year! This was impacted by my new ability to do many of the Open workouts as prescribed rather than scaling them to be easier.

When ECHF purchased an InBody Scanner, another level of fitness tracking became available. This device can determine a person's muscle mass, body fat mass, BMI, and percent body fat. In August 2017, I had my first InBody scan. It indicated that the amount of fat in my body was disproportionate to my overall weight/size. I was "skinny fat." What was I to do?

My first response was to just keep "showing up" and see what would happen over time. A year later, I did see a 2-lb. increase in muscle mass and a 1.7-lb. decrease in body fat. I decided to step it up and commit to working out at least three times a week with the goal of accelerating this pattern. It worked! In three months, I gained another pound of muscle and lost .6 lbs. of fat. Through all this time, I had not particularly changed my nutrition at all, eating whatever I wanted. I was aware that eating too much would cause a weight gain (and not due to muscle) and so tried to stay within my BMR of 1200 calories.

In October 2018, I decided to experiment with a change in diet while keeping to my 3-times-a- week training to see if there would be a measurable result. I began a diet that involved eating only meat, fat, and dairy… no sugar, no vegetables, no fruits, no carbs of any kind. Would this radical way of eating make a difference?

After only four weeks, I had lost 2.1% body fat with no loss of muscle mass! *So, in four weeks, I lost as much body fat as I had in 14 months of working out and eating whatever I wanted*. I continued with this way of eating, and an InBody scan after another six weeks showed an additional loss of 2.4 lbs. of body fat and a gain of 1.1 lbs. of muscle.

My InBody scan on February 16, 2019 (7 more weeks) showed another loss of 1.5 lbs. body fat and a gain of 1.3 lbs. of muscle. From the beginning of my carnivore eating and fitness consistency, I had gained 2.4 lbs. of muscle and lost 7.8 lbs. of fat! With those kinds of results, I decided to continue carnivore eating and consistently working out, but I stopped detailed tracking of my nutrition and workout regimen.

Then, significant changes occurred in March 2020. Gyms closed due to the Covid-19 pandemic. At first, the CrossFit gym I went to let members borrow equipment and work out in Zoom sessions. I did that for a little while but didn't like it, so I began working out by myself using the posted workouts from the gym. When the gym reopened, I decided to continue my at-home fitness regimen instead of going back. This meant canceling my gym membership and returning their equipment, so I needed a new plan.

I created a gym space in my home that included barbells and weights, a bench press rack, a rower, a treadmill, a universal machine, and other things like a plyo box, slamball, medicine ball, dumbbells, and kettlebells. Eventually, I added a pull-up bar and rings. I had the equipment but needed someone to program workouts for me.

That is when I began using the APEX At Home functional fitness program created by Bronson. So, although I didn't track nutrition, get body scans, or faithfully work out three times a week, I did continue to eat a primarily carnivore diet and worked out fairly regularly for the next two years.

By January 2022, I was curious about the result of my more casual approach to fitness over the past three years and decided to purchase a home InBody scanner to find out. I was quite surprised and pleased to discover that I had only lost about one pound of skeletal muscle mass and gained only 0.2% body fat. So, even without strict compliance with carnivore eating and intensive 3-day-a week exercise, I had maintained a good level of muscle mass (38%) and a level of fat that, while not ideal, is not nearly as much as it has been in the past.

A carnivore way of eating coupled with regular resistance exercise has yielded a level of fitness that allows me to do anything that I want to do. Fitness is freedom!

Mindset

Everything starts with how you think. Your perception and the reality you create for yourself affect your attitude, expectations, and eventual results.

If you begin this journey by establishing a positive mental focus, understanding what drives you, and knowing exactly how you're going to reach your goals, you cannot fail!

The rest of this book is pointless if you don't get your mind right. Tools and knowledge only go so far. You must have the mental fortitude to use them every day, no matter what.

"I have learned a great deal about nutrition and how our body uses the fuel provided to it. Bronson has presented us with a detailed plan of attack on how to transform our bodies, minds, and spirit.

I have learned more about how our bodies move and function for optimal fitness. My mind has been cleared of mental clutter and barriers to improving my fitness. My spirit has been lifted as I see and feel solid results from our simple plan.

I have learned that I can adapt my lifestyle, my diet, and my approach to nutrition in a positive way to reach the goals I have set for myself. I have learned that, despite my nearly complete and total failure to take care of myself physically all these years, I can improve my level of fitness, reverse adverse health conditions, and improve my quality of life through nutrition and exercise. No magic pills, no fitness gadgets, and no one is coming to save me except me." **- Jonathan Schiller**

Get in touch with your "Why"

Why are you doing it?

The most important question you can ask yourself is, "Why am I doing this?" I'm not talking about losing 10 pounds, getting back to your pre-baby weight, or even because your doctor said you need to. I'm talking about knowing what the changes you want to make will do for your everyday life and their impact on you and everyone in your life.

Your decision to get healthy has a much bigger impact than just losing some weight. What does it mean to you? How will your life change? What will you be able to do? Who will you inspire, and what kind of example will your effort provide for others?

Getting out of shape doesn't come by accident. It is a deliberate action, repeatedly producing a result. The law of inertia means that it will take MORE deliberate action with MORE consistency to reverse the momentum of your fitness and health and start moving in a positive direction.

When you're at the movies and the smell of popcorn and sight of people eating french fries and candy is all around you, your reason for staying true to your goals must be larger than the temptations around you.

The only thing that will keep you going is knowing why you're doing it. Your "why" has to be bigger than your "but".

Finding you're "Why"

No one wakes up in the morning and randomly decides to lose weight. Losing weight is a goal many people use after years of mental or physical trauma caused by poor health and physical ability. People want to lose weight due to feeling worthless, lack of independence, chronic pain, and illness. There is always a bigger reason than the weight itself.

You don't want to lose weight. You want what you think losing weight will do for your quality of life and mental health. It's the effect on how you live every day that matters, not how much you weigh.

Here are some signs that you've dug deep enough and found the real reason you want to change your life.

1. You can't think about it without getting emotional. When you find your "Why" it will make you angry, sad, give you hope, or fire you up! You shouldn't be able to have an unemotional conversation about your "Why".
2. Nothing is too inconvenient. The things you thought would be a challenge won't be nearly as tough. When you are in touch with your "Why", you don't let anything stand in your way.
3. You won't hear the noise. People don't like change. Many people in your life will try and keep you where you are. Not everyone is ready to do what you're doing. When you have a solid reason that drives you forward, no one will be able to stop you.

The 7 Levels of Why

Here is an exercise you can do to help get to the real reason you've started this journey. Be honest with yourself. No one is watching but you.

NOTE: This is NOT a five-minute exercise. It may take you a week to get through this. Dig deep, and don't let fear or embarrassment hold you back.

Q: Why do you want to _____? (fill in the blank with whatever you're goal or objective is.)

A: Because _____.

Q: Why is it important to _____? (Enter your answer from the preceding question.)

A: It's important because _____.

Q: Why is it important to _____? (Enter your answer from the preceding question.)

A: It's important because _____.

Q: Why is it important to _____? (Enter your answer from the preceding question.)

A: It's important because _____.

Q: Why is it important to _____? (Enter your answer from the preceding question.)

A: It's important because _____.

Q: Why is it important to _____? (Enter your answer from the preceding question.)

A: It's important because _____.

Q: Why is it important to _____? (Enter your answer from the preceding question.)

A: It's important because _____.

If you take the time to sit with these questions and dig deep to find the answers, you will come out with a new level of understanding and the power to reach your goals.

Your "Why" is the most powerful motivational tool you have. Don't lose it.

Pro-Tip

If you're struggling with identifying your "Why", start looking at the things you've been using as excuses for not doing what you know you should.

Your excuses are just your reasons in disguise.

- "I don't have time." is really "I need to make time and get better at organizing my life."
- "I'm too old." is really "I need to get healthy to be more independent as I get older."
- "I'm not a gym person." is really "I want to be an active person and need to improve my physical ability."

Every single excuse you can make is a reason you need to take action to improve your life!

How to set goals

Your "Why" will give you the drive and motivation to work hard. You still need to know what you're working for and where you're going. Goals give you a way to track and gauge your progress.

Be S.M.A.R.T

To make sure your goals are clear and reachable, each one should be

- Specific (simple, sensible, significant).
- Measurable (meaningful, motivating).
- Achievable (agreed, attainable).
- Relevant (reasonable, realistic and resourced, results-based).
- Time-bound (time-based, time-limited, time/cost limited, timely, time-sensitive).

SPECIFIC

Your goal should be clear and specific. Otherwise, you won't focus your efforts or feel truly motivated to achieve it. When drafting your goal, try to answer the five "W" questions:

- What do I want to accomplish?
- Why is this goal important?
- Who is involved?
- Which resources or limits are involved?

Example: I want to build muscle mass and improve my strength.

MEASURABLE

It's important to have measurable goals to track your progress and stay motivated. Assessing progress helps you stay focused, meet your deadlines, and feel the excitement of getting closer to achieving your goal. How will you know when you've reached the goal? A measurable goal should address questions such as:

- How much?
- How long?
- How fast?
- How heavy?

Example: I want to build 5 pounds of muscle mass and improve my strength to squat my body weight one time.

ACHIEVABLE

Your goal also needs to be realistic and attainable to be successful. In other words, it should stretch your abilities but remain possible. When you set an achievable goal, you may identify previously overlooked opportunities or resources that can bring you closer to it. An achievable goal will usually answer questions such as:

- How can I accomplish this goal?
- How realistic is the goal, based on other constraints, finances, or work schedule?

Example: I want to build 5 pounds of muscle mass and improve my strength to squat my body weight one time. I will do this by doing resistance training 3x a week and eating 1x my lean body mass in grams of protein per day.

Tip: Make sure you are setting goals for yourself. Don't be persuaded into saying you want to accomplish something just to make someone else happy or fulfill what you think someone else's desire for you is. Find out what makes you excited about your new life and go in that direction.

RELEVANT

This step ensures that your goal matters to you and aligns with other relevant goals. We all need support and assistance in achieving our goals, but it's important to retain control over them. So, make sure that your plans drive everyone forward but that you're still responsible for achieving your own goal. A relevant goal can answer "yes" to these questions:

- Does this seem worthwhile?
- Will this goal have a positive impact on my life?
- Does this match other efforts/needs?

Example: I want to build 5 pounds of muscle mass and improve my strength to squat my body weight one time. I will do this by doing resistance training 3x a week and eating 1x my lean body mass in grams of protein per day. Doing this will improve my daily energy and reduce my back pain.

TIME-BOUND

Every goal needs a target date to have a deadline to focus on and something to work toward. This part of the SMART goals criteria prevents everyday tasks from taking priority over your longer-term goals. A time-bound goal will usually answer these questions:

- When?
- What can I do six months from now?
- What can I do six weeks from now?
- What can I do today?

Example: In the next six months, I want to build 5 pounds of muscle mass and improve my strength to squat my body weight one time. I will do this by doing resistance training 3x a week and eating 1x my lean body mass in grams of protein per day. Doing this will improve my daily energy and reduce my back pain.

Now that's a goal you can build a solid plan from. What will your first goal be?

How to value your health

You are in your mid-forties or older. You are a good 25-35 lbs. over-weight, maybe more. You haven't done any real exercise in years. You think you eat well, or you know you don't, but there's some improvement to be made either way. You have high blood pressure, or you're insulin resistant. You've been told you're pre-diabetic, have high cholesterol, and are at risk for heart disease, a stroke, or worse.

Because you're overfat, unhealthy, and out of shape, you're always tired and never have enough energy to get through the day. You get stressed out easily. You have a hard time sleeping. Your bathroom adventures are legendary. You may have skin issues like eczema or psoriasis. Your joints and muscles are sore or ache all the time.

Following a nutrition and fitness program will help reverse all these issues.

You live with pain, discomfort, lack of sleep, stomach issues, skin irritations, medications, doctors' visits, treatments, and potentially life-threatening illnesses.

Here are a handful of the things you could consider when evaluating a health program.

- The education and experience of the coaches
- The effectiveness of the program itself
- Feedback from current clients
- The structure of the program and its ability to meet you where you are
- The program's components and how it addresses your problems
- Even the simple question. Will this program work for me?

All of these important factors and your biggest make-or-break question is, *"How much does it cost?"*

Why is the monthly cost of a fitness or nutrition program more important than joining that program and possibly saving your life?

Sure, you have a budget. You have obligations to take care of things to support your family and maintain your lifestyle. What happens to your family and lifestyle after you have a stroke or a heart attack?

Talking about money is a sensitive subject for people who don't understand the value of what they provide. As a health and fitness coach, it is my responsibility to help you see what you can do to live longer and have more freedom to do what you want to do with your life and your family.

When you use money, instead of what success in that program means for you and your family, as the reason to not start a program that you know will be good for you, you're selling yourself short.

Here are a few things to ask yourself if you find a program that will help you but you aren't sure you can afford it.

- How long have I been struggling to find a solution to my problems? If you've been looking for something that looks like it has all the pieces you need, how much longer can you afford to wait once you find it?

- Is it that much? An average, full service, health, and wellness program with coaching, nutrition, biometrics, and an effective fitness program will cost you $5-10 per day. How much is that lunch you eat out every day or that fancy coffee or couple of glasses of wine? Are those things helping you improve yourself?

- What does it cost if I get hurt or sick? Hospital bills, medications, doctor's visits, and lost work time can cost you thousands. Not to mention the restrictions placed on you and the activities you can participate in after an injury or serious health event.

- Do I know what to do? You decide to save money month to month and do it yourself. What do you do? How do you exercise? What do you eat? How do you measure performance? Are you doing the exercises properly so you don't get hurt? What's your overall plan for getting healthy, and how do you know if you're on track?

There are a ton of programs out there. Some may appeal to you more than others. Some will work better than others. There are old programs and new programs.

Health improvement programs are just like bars. There's more than one in every city. If you only look for the ones with the lowest happy hour prices, you know how that goes. You can have cheap, or you can have good, but you can't have both.

Fitness is health, not looks

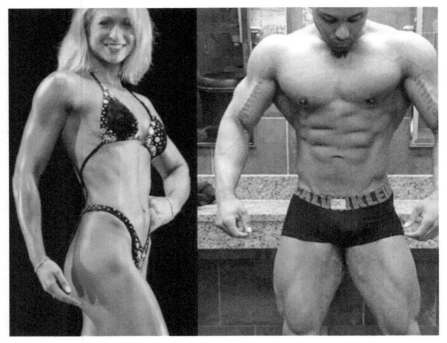

Figure 1 - Bodybuilders look healthy

What if I told you that neither of these people was healthy?

What if I told you that to get their bodies to look this way, they had to achieve an unhealthy mental attitude towards food and push their bodies to change beyond a functional need for muscle size and leanness?

Fitness is the physical representation of health. Being lean and muscular is not the same as being healthy. The visual depiction often idolized is not realistic. Nor is it a true indicator of health.

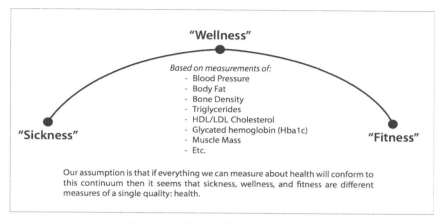

Figure 2 - Fitness Wellness Continuum

The woman pictured here had to shove food down her mouth that was boring. The stress of maintaining the rigid structure of show-prep pushed her to the max. She cried because of the stress and constant obsession she had to maintain over everything she ate. The hours spent working out and the single purpose she was working for actually set her back in her overall fitness. Her hormones were messed up, she was cranky, tired, and in her own words, "it was a horrible experience."

The man is now a functional fitness and boxing coach. He had been a bodybuilder for several years. He competed as a professional bodybuilder and, after a few years, realized how detrimental the sport was to his mental health and his body. The pressure to look a certain way was so high that it consumed his life, and he was out of balance in his priorities and health.

He realized how badly he was beating himself up and how unfit he was. In his words, "It's all about how you look. No one cares if you're healthy." He decided to change his focus and learn to improve his overall health and increase his fitness in all aspects of health. As a coach, he uses this experience to help others do the same.

We tend to look at athletes as the healthiest people. In many cases, they aren't. They look like they're in shape, so we equate that to mean healthy.

Athletes focus on a small portion of the fitness spectrum because each sport has a very specific demand on the body. It is not uncommon to have athletes specifically train their bodies to do things that intentionally put them in compromised health, higher risk of injury, and non-functional movement patterns.

Athletes train to perform a handful of specific actions. Yes, their bodies become and they look fit and healthy. However, our bodies perform various functions under different circumstances, environments, and stresses.

Just because someone has a fit look doesn't mean they have health. Health is a result of improving your body's ability to do work anywhere, in any circumstance. Improve these ten things, and you will see your quality of life improve dramatically.

Endurance: How long can you go?

Stamina: How long can you sustain a high level of effort?

Strength: How much weight can you move?

Flexibility: How well do your joints work?

Power: How much weight can you move quickly?

Speed: How quickly can you move?

Coordination: Can you feel and control complex movements?

Accuracy: Can you make your body do what you want it to?

Agility: Can you change direction efficiently?

Balance: Can you use your body unilaterally?

If you stop looking at the super "in shape" person and start looking at the little things you can do for yourself each day, you will see that even the smallest changes can quickly make a difference. If you follow the right plan, you can make big strides in as little as 90 days.

You can focus on simply improving your metabolism by reducing the crap you eat and doing more physical activity than you're doing now. You can start to get in shape and get healthy today.

Painting an old rusty broken car doesn't make it run any better. It's a lot of time and money spent on something you still can't use. In most cases, what you see on social media or in marketing content is not what you're after.

If your goal is to improve your daily life, your actions should match that goal.

- Nutrient Density
- Bioavailability
- Satiety
- Frequent movement at varying intensities
- Move weight often

It's your journey, don't look at other people and wish to be like them. They may be worse off than you are. Focus on your health and take it one step at a time.

Remember when fitness was fun

As a kid, exercise is a part of life, not something you do extra.

You stayed outside all day. You climbed around your treehouse, ran around the neighborhood, climbed fences and played tag, built a fort out of lawn furniture, and played cops and robbers. You dug holes in the woods to bury some imaginary treasure. After hours of playing, you never stopped moving. The last thing you wanted to hear was Mom or Dad yelling out the window for you to come in for the night.

Remember those days? Did you ever stop to think about how much exercise that was?

As a kid, you spent hours upon hours working out, and you never once thought of it as boring, tedious, or annoying. I bet you didn't equate the time you spent "playing" like work.

What happened? When did exercise become something you have to talk yourself into, a thing to be done as a last resort, or worse yet, something to be avoided?

You got older, you have more responsibilities, sure. The biggest thing that happened, though the method of exercise, changed. You are an adult now. You can't go running around your neighborhood building forts and climbing fences. That might end up in some interesting local police blotter reports.

Many activities done as "grownup playtime", things like rock climbing, hiking, or sports, take time and money, making them difficult to participate in regularly. What do you do? You join a gym or buy some fitness equipment that you can use at home.

By themselves, the "at-home" gym and the fitness club membership are great ideas, but they provide little direction or progress toward the goals you're trying to attain. While the accessibility and ease of use make you feel engaged in improving your fitness, there are some major gaps in the function and process these methods offer.

Playing with friends was one of the biggest reasons you did not think about how much you exercised as a kid. If you go to a regular gym now, can you name ten people you know personally at that gym? Name 3-5 that you work out with regularly if you can do that. (not someone you work out next to, but that you work out together). Chances are you can't. In most gyms, there is no community, no one to push you and make you want to do better.

A good fitness program builds a community that can share, motivate, and support. You should have other people doing the same things and going through similar challenges to cheer you on when you need it.

As a kid, there was always a mission or a plan. Whether catching the bad guy or hosting a tea party, you always knew what you were doing and why you were doing it. When was the last time you knew what you were going to do for a workout and how today's workout benefits you and affects the workout you do tomorrow? How about your overall plan for the next three months? Do you have a goal, and do you know what you need to do to achieve that goal? If you can answer yes to all of that, fantastic! Most people cannot.

The fitness club or "at-home" gym is a great tool. Unfortunately, these tools often don't come with instructions. One mark of a good fitness program is coaching and programming that helps you progress over time. It should be a training program with a purpose, a plan, and measurable performance. You should always have a coach whose sole purpose is to make you better. You should never have to wonder what you will do or be unsure if your program will help you meet your goals.

If you want to make fitness fun and enjoy the process of improving your quality of life, find a tribe and find a program or coach who can give you direction and help keep you on track. Feeling like a kid again is possible no matter how old you are.

Mindset shifts you need to make

You've decided to make some changes, but you don't know where, how, or what to do. Here are a few tips that will get you moving and give you a good foundation to build off and keep you going for a long, long time.

I've been a fitness professional for many years. As a coach, personal trainer, and former gym owner, I've seen thousands of people make changes to improve their quality of life. Some people succeed, others have limited success, and sadly many people don't stick with it for very long and never see the benefit.

Here are my tips for getting started and maintaining lifelong physical freedom.

It's a marathon, not a sprint

You've heard it before, but did you pay attention? Be patient if the goal is to be healthy, stay active, and maintain a high quality of life until you die. It took you years to get out of shape and unhealthy. It will take some time to get your health and fitness back.

Even if you're 65 years old and just getting started, you've got 15, 20, 25 years to work on yourself. Be patient.

One of the biggest challenges today is dealing with short-term gratification. Everything needs to be easy and quick. That's not how this process works.

The process of change fluctuates between overnight life-altering adjustments to slow, almost imperceptible changes. You have to be aware of this going in. Every day isn't going to be amazing. That's where the next tip comes in real handy.

Celebrate every success

Embrace the small wins, and you will keep the journey alive. Of course, this assumes you're setting goals along the way and keeping track of how you're doing.

Your progress can only be verified and celebrated by how far you've moved towards your goal. If you lose 1% body fat or learn a new exercise, how does that move you forward, and is that good? If it is, you can celebrate it.

Celebrating the little things along the way reminds you that the process is working and that you are making a difference in your life.

Celebrate positive health improvements, body changes, strength accomplishments, developing new habits, compliments from friends and family, and anything else that makes you feel good about yourself and what you're doing to improve.

Get help

Acknowledge that you have no idea what you're doing and get help. Find a Personal Trainer, join a gym with coaches who can help you, subscribe to an online fitness program, or get an online trainer or coach. You need consistent guidance and feedback from someone who knows how to get you where you want to be.

Improving your fitness and health is not DIY for most people. It's complicated and challenging trying to figure it out for yourself. There's so much information, and you do not know how to filter and apply what will work for you.

You will save time, money, setbacks, frustration, and most likely an injury or two by paying someone as soon as possible to help you get started. It is well worth the investment in your health. Long-term, it will still be less than what you'd pay the medical industry if you stayed unhealthy and worsened as you got older.

Build habits

Most people last longer and see more success by changing one or two things at a time. It's unrealistic to think you can make a massive shift and disruption to your lifestyle overnight.

Start small with something you can maintain until it becomes a natural occurrence. There are a couple of things you need to be aware of.

1. There are things you're doing that negatively impact your ability to improve. Sometimes stopping a habit is as important as starting one.
2. There will be something that you do not want to change. Doing that thing will be the biggest success on your journey.

Don't go from little physical activity to hitting the gym five days a week and completely altering your food choices. Start simple. Maybe go for a walk 3x a week or do two classes at the gym until you feel more comfortable and ready for more. Maybe stop adding cream and sugar to your coffee, or don't drink soda anymore.

Baby steps. Think about it. 1-year-olds aren't running. It's a process for them to learn and grow into. Right now, you are a 1-year-old in fitness and nutrition. Stop trying to run.

Find a tribe

Humans thrive on and need communal support. To stay sane, be reminded that you're on the right track and that success is possible. You need to find other people who are on the same journey. You will feed off their experiences, and they will feed off yours. You will help keep each other moving forward.

There are a few ways you can do this.

1. You can join a gym that has a group fitness program. They usually have very supportive and tight-knit communities.

2. You can subscribe to an online program with a group forum where subscribers can share and communicate.

3. You can join online forums that fit your personality or goals or choice of fitness method. There are thousands of FB groups, Reddit groups, etc. You can interact with other people who have the same challenges, questions, fears, and successes.

These are five things I recommend you take a really hard look at and figure out what you need to do mentally to prepare for. You have control. Be deliberate and consistent. Follow the process, and it will take you where you want to go. No shortcuts. They never work and often make things worse.

Stop using "Old" as an excuse

"I used to be able to...", "I can't do that...", or the really good one, "I don't need to go that hard anymore."

These are the common phrases I hear from people in the '40s, '50s, and '60s whenever I talk to them about improving their fitness.

I'm 50. I'm in good shape. I work hard to keep myself fit because it lets me do things I want to do. I never have to miss out on a life experience because I'm not physically fit enough to do it.

It's not about recapturing my youth. It's not about working out hard to be "hardcore". It is not about intensity for intensity's sake. It's about three things.

- Physical Freedom
- Self Confidence
- Independence

I've talked to many people who off-handedly discount their health based on past accomplishments and their perceived inability to reach those levels again. Halting your future by holding onto your past is such a depressing state of being.

Where you are today and what you could do to improve your health and fitness has nothing to do with what happened in the past. The whole idea of fitness is improving your ability to do work. Nothing says it needs to be compared to anything you've done before.

You are where you are, not where you were.

"I used to be able to squat 400 pounds. I can barely squat 200 pounds now before my knees start hurting." ....is NOT a reason to not work out. It's a reason you SHOULD be doing something to improve your ability to do things.

"I used to hit the gym hard and played soccer for years. Now I have a bad hip, or bad knees, or a bad back, or bad ankles....so I "can't" do anything to stay in shape anymore." ...This is an excuse, not a reality. You don't do anything because it may not be at the same performance level as it once was, making you feel old.

That's OK. You are older, not done.

You're older. Your body is changing. It takes longer and twice the work to build muscle. It takes longer to recover after working hard. You have to watch your nutrition more closely. Once you hit 40, TIME is working against you. The LAST thing you want to do is let it wear you down without a fight.

Starting a health and fitness routine should be challenging. If it weren't, it wouldn't help you improve. The act of exercising is something you do based on where you are right now. Not where you were 20 years ago. So you've had a hip or knee replacement. Get someone to help you work with that and get better. Learn how to push yourself for your health, not for the sake of your pride.

You'll never be 25 again. You may never have a six-pack. You'll probably never squat 400 pounds. You can enjoy more activities, have more energy, life, and vitality, and live a longer, more adventurous life.

Isn't that worth 3-5 hours a week? Isn't that worth paying more attention to what you eat? Isn't that worth asking someone for help?

How long is it going to take?

We're always in such a rush. We want everything right now. Our relationships with other people can't seem to survive the period of separation it takes to drive to work in the morning. We have to be in constant text, video chat, or messenger communication.

We need our entertainment delivered in the fastest way possible. If someone developed a retinal video implant where Netflix could stream video to our eyeballs, it would sell out in minutes. Fewer people are going to sporting events because it's easier and faster to just watch it on TV.

Unfortunately, this is also how people think of their fitness. *How fast will I get in shape? When will I get a 6-pack? How long will it take to lose the fat on my arms?* These are the most common types of questions I get asked.

This mindset is so flawed it's almost impossible to respond in a way that the person asking doesn't feel discouraged before they've even started. The first thing that needs to happen is a change in mindset.

Start by redefining what fitness is. Fitness is NOT being skinny. Fitness demonstrates health, movement, and engaging in physical activity without limitations. Fitness is handling what life throws at you on any given day.

Fitness is a state of being, NOT a destination. Being in shape is like being happy. You don't reach "happy", and then you're done.

Ask someone you think is in shape if they are in shape. Nine times out of 10, they'll say they still have work to do.

Once you understand that becoming fit is a series of habits created over time, then you'll start to understand that there is no real time frame you can put on it. You can set goals that will help you gauge your improvement but being "fit" is a process of constant improvement. You can start today and be more fit tomorrow.

Goal setting is important when you start on the road to fitness. Having a coach or mentor to keep you on track is also a key to success.

Whatever goals you set, here are some things to consider if you're wondering how long it will take to get there.

How long did it take you to get out of shape?

How old are you? How long has it been since you maintained an active lifestyle or worked out regularly? Have you been eating healthy or not? Many factors led to you being out of shape. None of them happened overnight.

What realistic expectation is there to get fit in any fraction of that time?

Here are some things that can help you have sustained success. Remember, moving closer every day is where you find success. Progress is the goal, whether it takes six months or two years.

How willing are you to work hard consistently over time?

It's not going to be easy. You have to make changes in your life. Your schedule, habits, activities, and time with people may have to change in one way or another.

That's not even taking the actual working out into consideration. You'll be sore, tired, and frustrated as you exercise and learn to work your body efficiently.

Can you remember why you're doing it and keep working hard consistently?

Food, food, food

You can't outwork a bad diet. It's that simple. Here's my basic nutrition guideline: Eat nutrient-dense, highly bio-available food that keeps you full as long as possible (satiating).

Ask yourself if the food you're eating is hurting or helping you reach your goals. If you don't know, I'd suggest starting to ask questions and learning as much as you can. There is more to it, and I highly suggest working with a professional to make sure you're doing it right.

Most important!

Quick is not the answer

Get over the fact that it will take time and effort. The worst thing you can do is try to shortcut the process by using gadgets, supplements, wraps, or something else that will supposedly help you "Lose weight in 60 days" or give you "3 secrets to lose fat.

That's it, folks. Eat the way nature intended and move your body as nature intended. Remember, fitness is a series of habits developed over time. Start small, get help, be patient.

How to get out of your comfort zone

You've heard it before.

"Get out of your comfort zone."

"The only way to grow is to get comfortable with being uncomfortable."

Here's the thing, sometimes it's hard to know when you're in your comfort zone or how to get out of it.

There are obvious limits to what you're comfortable with. I would expect bungee jumping off a bridge well outside your comfort zone. Did you know that something as small as not adding sugar to your coffee every morning could be more challenging and impactful on your life?

Getting outside your comfort zone is a decision to do something you don't want to do.

Think about that for a minute. Your desire to improve has to be strong enough to get you to do something that you know will be difficult. Growth and change require deliberate action. They don't happen by accident.

Are you in your comfort zone?

- Are you seeing progress?
- Do you feel like you've tried everything, but nothing changes?
- Are you stuck in a routine that you've gotten used to?
- Do you feel like there's more, but you aren't sure what to do?

These are all signs that you're stuck in a place that feels like you should be making progress, but you aren't doing enough to make real change happen. By definition, this is your comfort zone.

Get out of your comfort zone.

1. The first thing you should do to get out of your comfort zone is asking someone for help. Getting an objective point of view will give you ideas and help you see things that you wouldn't see on your own.

2. Identify one or two small, less intimidating, or life-adjusting things that you can start now. Habits are easy to form, and the smaller the activity, the more successful you'll be at building it into your lifestyle.

3. Don't procrastinate. Pick something to change and do it today. Right now. Immediately.

4. Tell some friends that you need support. Associate with other people who are also getting out of their comfort zones. Support them in their efforts. The more you can share the process with others, the better your chance of success.

Being comfortable isn't a bad thing. Living in a place of stagnant potential is depressing. Go make a positive change in your life.

Do you really want it?

Have you ever read something that made you stop and go, "Woah"? I don't remember where I read this, but I recently found it in my notes with a caption that said, "when you stop, you're not getting anywhere".

Here it is: "Obstacles and challenges are not put before you to keep you from your dream. They are put there to see if you want it."

Every time I read this, I get chills. I feel like I overcome a challenge every day.

Being an entrepreneur requires me to constantly live outside my comfort zone, do things I was never taught, and learn things in real time. The mistakes have been plenty, and the learning curve is steep. It's hard every day.

But I do what I can to take a step forward each day because my dream is to help people get healthy and experience life as much as possible. I want to make a difference in the world, and my comfort zone isn't going to keep me from doing that.

You have struggles and challenges every day too. Not only do you have your family and jobs, but you have your own goals and dreams of things you want to accomplish.

When it comes to your health and fitness, you know what you need to do and what you should do. In many areas, you may even want to do those uncomfortable things like meal prep on the weekends, get up early for a class, or stretch on the living room floor while watching tv.

When it comes time to decide one way or the other, the thought process isn't really about what you will do or what's convenient, easy, or difficult. It's only about one thing.

How badly do you want to see a change in your life?

Whenever you sit on the couch instead of stretching on the floor, you're reinforcing movement in the opposite direction of your goals.

Every time you sleep in or make an excuse not to work out, you decide to stay right where you are.

Every time you have "just one drink", you're telling yourself and everyone around you that you aren't serious about getting in shape. You want that drink more than you want to fix your metabolism.

This may sound a little harsh. That's OK. It's not my job to make people feel good about making decisions that hurt them.

That's what makes this statement so powerful

Obstacles and challenges are not put in front of you to keep you from your dream. They are put there to see if you want it.

There are no real obstacles or challenges for someone who truly wants something bad enough. When you want it badly, you'll find a way to make it happen. What do you need to want more physical freedom, strength, vitality, and happiness in your life?

What's Your "Why"?

Whatever you need to do to get excited about improving your health, go do it!

Listen to this. Listen.

NOTHING is stopping you, but you.

- You can be fit.
- You can be strong.
- You can lose body fat.
- You can feel great about yourself again

Your Freedom is Your Choice.

Get long-lasting results

You want to be fit, active, and full of life well into your later years. That's why you're interested in improving your fitness and health. You want long-term solutions, not something that will get you a 6-pack in 6 weeks and then has you back in fat clothes six weeks later.

You're looking for a program that will give you results you can take to your grave.

Let's talk about the two biggest mistakes people make when they get started walking the road of self-improvement.

Have a plan

Too many people get on the Internet and try the "I'll ask 20,000 people what the best option for me is" method of starting a program… Think about that for a minute.

You're going to ask random strangers what's best for you. That's NOT the same as having a plan.

What is a plan? A plan is a set of information that includes:

- Where you are now, and how you got there
- Where you want to get to, when, and why
- What are the lifestyle factors that will affect your adherence and ability to follow the plan
- How you evaluate if the plan is working
- What is the process for adjustment if a change is needed

Does that look the same as what you would get off a random "WHAT'S THE BEST WAY FOR ME TO LOSE BELLY FAT" post in a Facebook group??

To develop a solid, realistic, and effective plan, you need a proven program that gives you all the pieces to the puzzle.

What happens when you start putting in the work but don't have a plan or a guide to making the work mean something?

It's so much more effort. Even if you're good at what you do, you WILL miss things if you just run with an idea before you take the time to consider the impact and possible courses of action. You will have to double back and re-do work. You'll generally work like a mad man who has no idea what he's doing. In many ways, you don't. How could you? You don't have a plan. Consider this. You aren't an expert on health, nutrition, or mindset. If you can't just wing it in something you're good at, how could you possibly be successful with your health?

It takes a lot of extra time. If you want to lose 10% body fat in 3 months, but you waste time trying five different methods because they didn't work in the first week, why did you set a three-month goal? Every time you change from one method to another without knowing, 1. how it fits into your plan (if you have one) and 2. what the intended results are, you're adding to the time it will take to achieve the changes you want to see.

You can do more harm than good. This is a supercritical factor when it comes to your health and fitness. Every time you have a setback, it creates more work, increases the time to your goal, and raises the risk of another setback. Here are a few things people have to deal with when they rush forward without a plan or try different things they "think" will work.

- Injuries
- Fat loss stalls
- Loss of lean mass (muscle)
- Setbacks in physical performance
- Frustration and lack of consistency
- In the worst cases, people have seriously messed up their hormones or reverted to a worse state of health that required medical intervention.

Chances of failure are way more likely. Considering everything I've just laid out, is it any surprise that you have a greater chance of overall failure? Without a plan, you have no direction, leading to frustration and a lack of consistency.

Many people jump from program to program, online routine to online routine, or diet to diet (see where this is going??) without seeing any progress.

They live a life of futility, never realizing their full potential.

Don't try everything all the time

When you don't start with a plan, you have no idea what will work, how to tell if it's working, or how long to wait to see if it works.

I see and hear it ALL THE TIME. "I started keto a few weeks ago, and I do not see any results. Should I try Intermittent Fasting to lose fat faster?"

And…"I did Paleo for a year, and I felt a lot better, but I couldn't lose any weight, so I went keto and gained weight after a couple of months, so now I'm trying Protein Sparing Modified Fasting to see if that works."

Or… "Do I need to add more cardio to my routine? I do CrossFit 3x a week, yoga 2x a week, and walk my dog 3 miles every day….?"

Every method and protocol has different expected times to see changes. Each of them requires a different level of detail and commitment to maintaining. Some are very sustainable. Some are in no way meant to be long-term solutions.

How are you going to know which one is right for you? What to expect, or how to keep it going long enough to see results if you don't have a coach and a plan to follow?

Everyone starts as a beginner before they become advanced enough to be self-sustaining.

Nutrition or Fitness, you CAN NOT shortcut that process.

A beginner is a blank slate with no good foundation physiologically, in their central nervous system, or psychologically. Just about ANY added stimulus will create some kind of positive change. Just by taking consistent action, a beginner will improve.

And then they won't.

There will be a reduction in the amount of progress a beginner sees from their work. They will eventually move into an intermediate area that requires introducing a higher level of slightly more complex methods and protocols to get the response from their body that they're looking for.

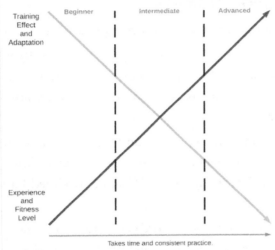

Figure 3 - Training Effect and Adaptation

Just the sort of things a coach can help them figure out.

This process continues the closer a person gets to what is called their "genetic potential". The closer you get to the upper limit of what your body can do, the more deliberate and exacting you have to be in how you work to get your body to make even the smallest changes. This advanced level is rare, and your normal 9-5 Jane and Joe will probably never get there.

That's ok. You don't need to get there to be functionally fit and have a super high quality of life.

As I said, you CAN NOT shortcut this process

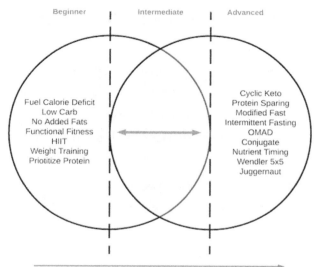

Figure 4 - Beginner to Advanced Progression

You need to be keto-adapted and metabolically healthy before implementing a Cyclic Ketogenic Diet.

You need to be able to Squat and Deadlift correctly under a good amount of weight before you try to follow Wendler 5×5.

Ensure you're getting adequate protein before worrying about nutrient timing.

Where do you fit in the grand scheme of your journey? Are you a Beginner or Intermediate?

To give you a reference. I've been in the fitness business for over ten years. I'm Intermediate in most aspects, a beginner in a few, and advanced in even less.

There is no real timeline. Everyone is different. The best judge of where you are and what you need is objective and should not be made by you looking at yourself in the mirror.

Get an expert to guide you.

The secret to making progress

The secret to building muscle, reducing inflammation, and improving your quality of life is being honest with yourself and accepting the changes that facilitate the progress you want to achieve.

Your goals can only be reached by doing things differently than you have in the past.

Take a second and think about that.

If you want things to be different, you have to do different things.

Changing what you do requires a level of honesty with yourself that will be uncomfortable. Getting outside your comfort zone is more than just the physical aspects of fitness or the mental effort of cutting out sweets. You have to be transparent with yourself and understand your choices every day.

Self-evaluation and learning to identify appropriate changes will keep you moving forward and help you avoid stalls and plateaus.

I'm going to break down how to evaluate key fitness and nutrition components. You can follow this guide when looking for ways to improve your results. Only you will know if you're doing what it takes in each area. Don't lie to yourself or make justifications.

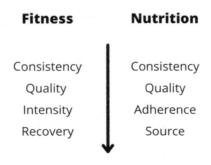

Fitness   **Nutrition**

Fitness	Nutrition
Consistency	Consistency
Quality	Quality
Intensity	Adherence
Recovery	Source

Sustained Progress

Figure 5 - The process of self-evaluation

How to evaluate your fitness

The four areas that affect how well you improve your fitness are:

- Consistency
- Quality of movement
- Adequate Intensity
- Sufficient Recovery

It is impossible to maintain success with inconsistent effort. Long breaks between workouts, cutting workouts in half, or skipping things you don't "feel" like doing will never get you where you want to go.

Always focus on quality movement before speed or weight. If you improve the movement, you will be able to increase the speed and weight safely. The added intensity will have more benefit when the movement is correct.

You need to push yourself. It should be uncomfortable. I'm not saying painful or unsafe. You can make it challenging in a few different ways.

- Move better
- Increase the skill needed (use a more complicated version of a movement)
- Increase weight
- Increase speed

You should feel like you pushed yourself as hard as possible after every workout.

You cannot progress towards something you've never done without the work also being something you've never done.

Don't get me wrong. I know you work hard. Have you ever thought you could have done more work?

- After the workout, have you thought you had a little more in the tank?
- After a workout, have you stayed and done the accessory work or cool-down your coach has given you?

Improvements in physical performance happen during periods of rest. If you are not allowing yourself to recover, you are always working in the wrong direction. Take a day or two off each week. Get more sleep. Spend a day or two just stretching, getting a massage, or doing something to help your recovery.

Are you consistent, trying to move well, working hard enough, and resting appropriately?

Only you can answer those questions.

How to evaluate your nutrition

The four areas that impact how well your nutrition works for you are:

- Consistency
- Quality of nutrition (whole vs. processed)
- Adherence to the plan
- Source of nutrition (effect on body and results)

When you are trying to get out of debt with your health, every choice matters. Like fitness, being inconsistent will stall your progress faster than anything else. Long-term improvement is when small choices build up over time and lead to big results. Remember, the goal is not perfection. Consistently make more choices that move you forward.

Whole food choices will always be better for you than anything with an ingredient label. Process foods are less nutrient-dense, more inflammatory, and higher in calories. If you want to make progress without any question about how good a food option is for you, start focusing on real, natural, whole food.

Common ingredients in processed foods that could hold you back

- Unlisted sugar/carbs (There are 90+ names for sugar)
- Seed oils (sunflower, corn, grapeseed, soy, etc.)
- Soluble fibers (xanthan gum, acacia gum, guar gum, etc.)

Processed foods have one benefit, convenience. When you choose convenience, you are sacrificing nutritional benefits. There may be times when that is needed. Only you can determine if it's a choice you're willing to make consistently.

Your macros matter. There is a reason to set macro goals and stick to them as closely as possible. Adherence to your macro plan will greatly impact your success.

- Are you tracking everything?
- Are you entering accurate info?
  - If you have to choose between different but similar items, always choose the food with the lowest protein and highest fat.
- Are you paying attention to ingredient labels or just looking at the number of carbs listed?
- Always use Total Carbs!

Here's a tricky one. Whether food is whole or processed, it may harm your health or slow your progress. Is it worth keeping in your life if it's holding you back?

Dairy is a great example of this. I know for me, cheese makes it harder to lose fat. It affects my digestion, and if I have too much overtime, I will stall. Maybe you've been stalled for a while. Are you drinking shakes made with milk proteins? How much cheese are you eating?

You may have issues with some meats, or some vegetables may cause an adverse reaction. Everyone is different. You have to pay attention to what is happening in your body. If you are not making the progress you want, it could be something you're eating, **even if that food is considered to be generally healthy.**

Are you consistently eating whole food, sticking to your macros, and listening to your body?

Only you can answer those questions.

It's only hard if you think it's hard

Taking care of your mind and body is a crucial aspect of living a happy life, being productive, and giving your family what it needs from you.

With all the things you have to deal with and the weight of responsibility on your shoulders, sometimes you sabotage your success and happiness. Little things creep in that keep you from living your best life and positively influence others.

Here are three things you may be doing to make your life harder.

- Complaining is stupid. It's not fun, and it's a mental exercise in futility that just makes people around you feel bad. It's a negativity virus.
- Making excuses is also a waste of time. The problem needs to get fixed, period.
- Comparing ourselves to others is the ultimate red herring. Nothing will steal your happiness faster than comparing yourself to someone else.

I'm not going to go too deep on these. Nothing about these three things should surprise anyone. Here's the real question. When was the last time you did some self-reflection to see if you may be doing one of them?

Have you felt defeated, discouraged, or like you're just spinning your wheels and nothing you do makes a difference? In many cases, those are signs that you've let negativity creep in, and you're missing the good stuff happening all around you.

It's easy to get into a pattern of behavior and not be aware you're doing any of these things. When you're dealing with the frustrations of life, you can forget that failure is an opportunity to improve and learn from the experience.

How do you get out of a negative rut? How do you keep yourself in a positive frame of mind as much as possible? Here are three things you can do to help your mindset and attitude work wonders on your health and overall lifestyle.

- Exercise will increase your body's ability to handle stress. It helps your brain process and manage external stimuli better and gives you the energy to function at a higher level for longer in a day. You can significantly improve your mental health by increasing your physical activity.
- Find a tribe that will give you the positive energy and accountability you need. Don't hang out with miserable people. Hang out with people who will give you crap for being a grouch.
- Set a goal and work your butt off to accomplish it. It doesn't matter what the goal is. It can be fitness, nutrition, sport, or paper mache related. Just go do the work to accomplish something and succeed in reaching your goals. Working towards a goal is, by definition, empowering and creates positivity and a growth mindset in you and those around you.

Yes, I want you to get in shape and eat right. Yes, I want you to live a long life and be strong through it. What good does any of that if you're stuck in a negative mindset most of the time?

Setting an example

If you're a parent, you know how scary it can be watching your children imitate the things you do and say. Their ability to absorb and reflect our mannerisms, attitudes and facial expressions can be eerie.

As a parent, you have to be aware of what you do and say around your kids. Watching you impacts their actions, decisions, and thought processes.

With that in mind, what are the lessons you most want to teach your kids? What do you think will help them the most in life? Is there a specific character trait, attitude, mindset, or philosophy you want them to live by in their adult years?

How do some of these sound?

- Work hard and become a leader
- Anything worthwhile takes time
- If it were easy, anyone could do it
- There's no elevator. Everyone has to take the stairs
- Every cloud has a silver lining
- Failure is an opportunity to learn and do better the next time
- Without failure, there can be no success
- Positivity is contagious
- A negative mindset will never give you a positive life
- Always start with why you want something
- Keep your dream alive
- The only competition is with yourself
- No one succeeds by themselves
- Without a coach or mentor, you're wasting time
- Learn from other people's mistakes
- Progress happens in little steps
- A bat never swung is ball never hit

- Your attitude determines your altitude
- Surround yourself with lions or get eaten with the sheep
- If you want to soar with the eagles, stop hanging around with chickens
- Motivation is directly related to how badly you want something, so want something badly

This list can go on and on and on….

These ideas and thoughts permeate through a person's effort to improve their health and fitness. The challenges and commitment it takes to change one's lifestyle force them to work through many situations where these come into play.

Engaging in the process of self-improvement brings obstacles in scheduling, money, dealing with other people, being coached, following a plan, staying committed, being positive, and focusing on the goals you've set.

Our kids see it all.

They don't necessarily know what goes on at your job or what you do in your social time. But, when you set a goal to change your lifestyle, it comes home with you like nothing else in your life.

They see the challenges you face and how you deal with them.

They see when you decide to do nothing and when you commit to doing what it takes.

You're setting an example for your kids to model one way or another. Choose carefully.

Why coaching should matter to you

Anytime someone wants to learn something new, they go to a place, physical or virtual, where someone with more knowledge will teach them. You see it in all aspects of life.

Music lessons, Dog training, learning a second language, computers, and knitting have resources people use to get guidance on how to perform the tasks they want to perform and improve their skills.

What if I told you that fitness and nutrition were no different?

No one is born with the knowledge and skill to play the guitar or work out and eat properly. Yet, for some reason, millions of people worldwide spend billions of dollars at gyms and on nutrition programs while having no idea what they're doing.

Too many people find a 6-week workout plan on a fitness website and run to the gym to get ripped or buy a "Lose 10 pounds in 10 days!" meal plan only to fail, feel like crap, and quit. Granted, for some people, it may work some of the time. But most people don't see any results at all. Without a personalized training plan, they fail.

Many factors go into building a program so that each person doing it will see success and at the same time make it work no matter the fitness level or lifestyle of the person doing it.

Each person has different goals and different starting points. Most people don't know how to...

...Build a fitness routine

...Correctly perform movements

...Evaluate and modify the program for improvement.

...Choose food that will heal them

For example, here are a few things to consider when improving your health and fitness.

- What are scaling and modification?
- How does progressive overload work?
- How can you benefit from super-compensation?
- What is hypertrophy, and how do you balance it with max effort work?
- When do you do accessory work?
- How important is myofascial release to the recovery process or muscle growth?
- When is the best time to stretch? What kind of stretching is best?
- Why is structural power transfer so important?
- What is transferability in movement?
- How important are nutrient density and bioavailability?
- What foods are the most satiating?
- How to use food to manage oxidative stress and inflammation?
- What are anti-nutrients?
- How much fiber do you need?
- How much protein does it take to build muscle?

These are some things that someone developing a well-rounded program should understand. Trust me. There's a lot more where that came from.

Remember how I said that fitness was just like the other things that people could learn and do?

It isn't.

Health is MORE complicated than all of them. Most of the skills people pay someone to teach them are rote skills. They are the same for everyone, and learning them is a matter of practice and memorization of repeated patterns.

Fitness and nutrition use the same principles for everyone, but the application to each person is completely different. Every person has a different body makeup, physical history, genetic profile, goals, and lifestyle. It is near impossible to make any single plan work the same for everyone.

You need to get a coach to guide you through the process. It's also why many people don't even consider getting help. It's too overwhelming, and they feel they'll never understand it all, so following a pre-packaged 6-Week "Get Jacked" program off the Internet is more attainable.

Except it doesn't work. At-home video workouts, high-tech spin bikes in the living room, 10-day detoxes, or cabbage soup diets by the millions, and Americans are still the most unhealthy people in the world.

The solution?

Find a coach.

A coach will walk you through the process by telling you what you need to do. You don't need to learn everything there is to know about health and fitness. You just need to do what the coach says and learn the pieces that apply to you.

A coach has done all the brain work for you. They are your supplemental source of knowledge. You don't have to learn about the human body, movement, nutrition, etc. They've done it for you.

Finding a coach gives you so many things that put you way ahead of anyone doing it on their own. You get:

- Personal guidance and direction
- Training on how to get the most of your program
- Progressive development
- Accountability
- Progress checks and adjustments
- Evaluation and correction
- Safety controls and training

Without a coach, you get:

- A gym to work out in
- Random short term workout plans
- Millions of people on social media
- Instagram "Fitness Professionals" you can follow
- The latest diet from a magazine you got at the grocery store

Which one looks like the more cost-effective and time-saving option for you?

Health and Quality of Life

I want this book to do a few things. One of them is to help you understand what it means to be healthy. There is an overriding theme I want you to keep in the back of your mind as you go through the rest of this book.

If you focus on building, improving, and growing, you'll have less time to worry about what you're cutting and removing from your life.

Improving your metabolic function is the foundation for improving your quality of life.

Health and living your best life isn't about getting skinny. It's not even about eliminating the dozens of illnesses or diseases millions of people deal with every day.

Those things will take care of themselves if you focus on the real issue.

"I've added fitness into my routine in the past year and a half. I started just following videos on YouTube but have switched over to Apex Training and now have an online coach that is available to answer any questions. I love the variety of the workouts, and the functional fitness aspect, which is important at my age. I want to age gracefully, being able to get up and down and be independent as long as possible. I've gained muscle and lost fat, and most importantly improved my bone mass." - **Kim C**

Your metabolism is your health

"I wish I had your metabolism."

"I just need to speed up my metabolism."

"If I eat many small meals throughout the day, I'll have a faster metabolism."

Have you ever heard or even said something like this? Do you equate your metabolism to how fast you can burn off a boston cream donut?

Unfortunately, there's a lot more to it than that.

Metabolism is more than just the fuel-burning process. Your metabolism is ALL your bodily processes. It is what all of your biological functions do for you to live.

Metabolism is the processing of nutrients in your body to sustain life. Your body manages two core processes that encompass a whole bunch of stuff.

- Catabolism – the breakdown of molecules to obtain energy and other resources
- Anabolism – the synthesis of compounds needed by the cells to function

You are a machine. You need fuel (fat/carbs). Your body breaks down what you eat to provide that fuel.

The other thing that you need is for your machinery to function properly. What you eat also provides the building blocks (protein) to ensure that each part of that machine works like they're supposed to.

Think about it this way. You're tearing things apart to use them as fuel, or you're putting things together so the machine (your body) can be more effective at tearing things apart to be used as fuel.

See the circular effect here?

When I talk about speeding up your metabolism, I'm not talking about fuel burn. I'm talking about increasing the efficiency of how your body functions. More efficiency could mean more fat burn. It could also mean faster recovery from strenuous activity or less inflammation due to stress relief on a particular system in the body. The potential benefits of improving your metabolism go far beyond plain old fat loss.

What can you do to improve your metabolism?

- Eat whole foods and cut out the crap. The more extra work your body has to do to get nutrients from your food, the less efficient it can run itself.
- Significantly reduce carbs. The more carbs you eat, the more work your body has to do to get anything out of them. Carbs add stress and make your body work harder than it needs to. (*More on this later or skip to the Nutrition Section of the book.*)
- Exercise. Give your body a reason to be more efficient. What do you think will happen if you sit around all day and don't make your body demand performance?
- Sleep. Give your body time to work and repair. Sleep and recovery optimize your progress in healing and strength.

Fitness is the physical representation of how well your body functions. The more fitness you have, the better your body functions, the more healthy you are.

What would happen if you improved your metabolism?

- Fat loss
- Fewer aches and pains
- Shorter recovery time
- Strength gains
- Reduced bowel issues
- Skin conditions may go away

- Better sleep
- Reduction in auto-immune symptoms
- Reduced symptoms of insulin resistance
- Healthier arteries
- Lower blood pressure
- Lower heart rate

Go ahead and speed up your metabolism. I dare you!

Do more work and live more life.

Have you ever told someone to "get to work"?

What is work? How do you "do" work? How does it have anything to do with my health?

How to define work

The scientific definition of work is, $W = Fd$ (Work = Force x distance)

Moving an object any distance requires some application of force greater than the weight, inertia, and other variable resistances affecting that object. This principle applies to many aspects of our everyday life. You could say that most people define work as simply "getting things done".

How people do work

A computer programmer goes to her job every day. She sits in a chair, walks around the office, she uses her cognitive faculties to accomplish her daily tasks.

A nurse goes to the hospital and walks around for 10 hours helping patients, moving people around in beds, and dealing with high levels of stress throughout his shift.

A stay-at-home mom is always on the job. She must be mentally quick, physically active, and handle a million tasks. She has the most demanding clientele in the world, and only the best will suffice.

Why work is important

Here's a secret that many people in the fitness world won't tell you.

Successful fitness programs are NOT designed to help you lose fat, get a six-pack, or "get ripped."

Seriously, they aren't. Besides, if your goal is to get a six-pack, you aren't looking for fitness. You're looking for a six-pack.

If "getting ripped" is the driving force behind your desire to workout, there are many places you can go and many products that can help you get there. But, your fitness will be a secondary concern, if it's a concern at all.

Successful fitness programs focus on increasing your capacity to do work.

Your body's ability to do work is directly relevant to your ability to perform at your job, in your home, and doing daily activities. If you are limited in how much work you can do, you hit a wall, and things go downhill from there. You feel tired. You can't concentrate. You need to take longer breaks. Less work gets done.

Basing your fitness program on increasing your ability to do work is important because it is the foundation for everything you do.

With better fitness, everyone can be more alert, have more energy throughout the day, handle stress, sleep better, get more done in less time, and generally feel better and be more efficient in everything they do.

Fitness has nothing to do with how you look. It has everything to do with how much work you can do.

Guess what??? As you increase your ability to do work, you also benefit from fat loss, muscle gain, a smaller waist, reducing clothing sizes, and gaining the appearance of fitness.

As you increase your fitness, you will look more fit.

Chasing the appearance of health rarely achieves health.

Boost your immune system

There is a lot of information available on preventative measures for viruses and diseases. Discussing what safety measures are effective or appropriate has become a very common and volatile topic. Unfortunately, most of the US population lives in poor metabolic health and compromised immune systems.

As a population, we aren't putting ourselves in the best position to deal with any sort of biological adversity.

- Almost 50% of the US population is obese.
- 45%, more than 58 million people, are Pre-diabetic or Diabetic.
- 24% of Americans have to deal with Arthritis.
- 33% of people have High Blood Pressure.

What impact will a virus have on a population already living in a state of chronic inflammation and poor metabolic health, combined with a sedentary lifestyle and a diet devoid of adequate nutrition?

When you're starting at ZERO, everything becomes a net negative.

There is never a 100% solution to combating any virus or disease. All you can do is put yourself in the absolute best position to deal with it when it happens.

You need to start doing this stuff ASAP! Here are five things you can do to boost your immune system.

Increase your muscle mass

Muscle plays a vital role in maintaining your body's ability to heal and repair. Low muscle mass is linked to a significant reduction in immune response and recovery times in viral infections, cancer treatment, etc.

Two things you can start doing right now to increase your lean mass.

- Eat more protein. Your body must have protein to keep you functioning properly.
- Start weight training. Muscle won't grow until it needs to. You have to stimulate growth by using your muscles.

Muscle is required to provide movement and physical freedom. If you don't feed or train your muscles, they won't do what your body needs them to do. Your physical ability will be limited, and your immune system will also be compromised.

Reduce inflammation

Chronic inflammation is the body's response to being forced to do things it doesn't want to for long periods. Short-term inflammation is part of the immune system's function. It tells the body something is wrong and triggers the healing process.

Chronic inflammation occurs when something repeatedly and consistently aggravates your body and attacks its systems. This aggravation changes inflammation from a useful function of the immune system to a source of damage and injury to the organism it's affecting.

Think of a small cut on your arm. At first, it's red, and the skin gets a little puffy. That's inflammation. What happens if you keep cutting yourself in the same spot every day? Will it ever heal? Will it get worse or infected? Will the inflammation spread?

The biggest source of chronic inflammation for most people is processed food. It's not natural, your body doesn't like it, but you keep eating it, meal after meal after meal. It affects your whole body and puts everything into a state of chronic inflammation.

Every bite of food you take that comes from a box and has an ingredient label longer than the Bill of Rights is just another cut over and over again.

Eating food as close to its natural state as possible is the best way to ensure the highest levels of nutrition and the lowest amount of toxicity and inflammation to your body.

Making a move to whole foods is one of the most significant changes you can make in your life, and it will let your body do its job to heal you from disease and sickness.

Improve mitochondrial function

Mitochondria are the cellular engines that make everything in your body function. If they aren't healthy, you aren't healthy.

Mitochondria are responsible for fueling and driving everything your body does, including managing the immune system. There are three things you can do to improve the health and performance of your mitochondria.

- Reduce Inflammation. Another way you can reduce inflammation is by increasing your sleep time. Sleeping is critical to healing and letting your body focus its energy on staying healthy.
- Give them better fuel. Mitochondria love to burn fat. Ditch the carbs. Fat is more energy-dense. It has nine calories per gram to burn. Carbs only have 4. It burns cleaner (fat generates less oxidative stress and free radical byproducts, which increase cancer risk), and there is an endless supply available.
- Make them work - Mitochondria are the powerhouses of physical activity. They get more efficient at producing energy when you ask them to do it. Vary the length and intensity of your workouts, so your energy production improves no matter what activity you do.

Support anabolic processes

The functions of your body that build muscle, heal, and recover are called anabolic processes. How do you give your body the support it needs to maintain your health and immunity?

- Reduce Inflammation. If your body doesn't have to keep trying to heal the same cut over and over, it can keep you healthy and be ready for anything new that it has to deal with.
- Start weight training. The more muscle you have, the stronger your body will be. Muscle is the organ of longevity and
- Eat more protein. I can't say this enough.
- Get more sleep. Sleep is when your body does most of its anabolic work because Testosterone and Human Growth Hormone are at their highest levels. Muscle protein synthesis builds and repairs muscle and tissue during sleep without much interference. Sleep is very, very important.

All of the major health issues in the United States are a symptom of the unhealthy lifestyle, chronic stress and inflammation, and poorly functioning metabolism of the average person today.

If you do all of the above, you will lose body fat, a big indicator of metabolic health. When you stop the chronic inflammation give your body the material and time to heal and function, you'll start to see some amazing things happen.

Improve your metabolic function, and you'll be much better prepared to fight off and recover from viruses than ever before.

Increase your energy

Chronic fatigue is one of the biggest reasons people try to make lifestyle changes. I know it was an issue I dealt with before changing my nutrition and exercise. I hated that low energy feeling, being lethargic throughout the day, getting to that 2:00 time in the afternoon just wanting to drop everything and take a nap.

There are a few things to keep in mind when talking about energy. Think about your energy levels like gas in a car. There are a handful of things that affect the performance and condition of an engine. In that context, you have to consider,

- The availability of the gas because an empty tank of gas doesn't work well.
- The available amount is how much you have stored or need to eat.
- The efficiency of how you burn it because the performance of the engine matters
- The condition of the vehicle and how often, and how well it's maintained.

The first thing to understand about energy is where it comes from. There are two things your body uses for fuel; Carbohydrates and Fats. No, I didn't forget Protein, it's not fuel, but we'll cover that later. While fat and carbs can provide energy to your body, they are processed differently, stored differently, and produce different results.

Slow vs. Fast fuel burn

The first way fat and carbs are different is that they have different amounts of energy by quantity. Fat has nine calories of energy per gram and carbs have four calories per gram. That means you get a longer fuel burn per gram of fat than per gram of carbs. Fat lasts longer and burns slower.

Fat is a better option for fuel because it requires less replenishment overall. You can have over 2x as much energy even if you eat a lower quantity of food. You get more consistent energy throughout the day without spikes and crashes. The slow, steady usage of fuel keeps things even all day long.

Clean vs. dirty burn

I covered this a little in the chapter on improving your immune system. Carbs burn hot. Fats do not. Since we're using gas in your car as the analog for fueling your body, think of carbs like an octane booster and fat like regular gas. You can use a ton of octane booster to make your engine run. It's going to cost a lot, you'll need to refill the tank more often, and it will burn up your fuel system.

All fuel processed by your body generates something called oxidative stress. Think of oxidative stress like the carbon build-up that your engine produces when it runs. Too much oxidative stress for a long period is bad for your body. It is the root cause of chronic inflammation and disease.

Burning carbs generates more oxidative stress than burning fats. The increase in oxidative stress creates a diminishing return on the energy you get. More interference equals worse results. The more dependent on carbs you are for energy, the more stress and less usable energy you get.

Store a little or store a lot

Do you like eating six times a day? Are you crashing and burning a few hours after every meal? Your energy source is running out faster than you can replenish it.

Your body stores around 400g - 500g of glycogen in the liver, muscle tissue, and blood. That's around 2000 calories of energy. Since that's the average caloric intake of most people, it's easy to see how you have to keep fueling up repeatedly.

On the other hand, Fat is almost limitless in how much can be stored. For example, a woman who is 150lbs at a healthy, 23% body fat has 32lbs of fat on her body. That's 130,635 calories of energy she has stored that are ready to go as needed.

Another reason why training your body to use fat is a more efficient way to improve your daily energy and performance.

Improve your performance

If you love your car, you get a regular tune-up, replace parts, and make sure it's in good running condition. Keeping your car in good shape helps you get the most out of its performance, keep good gas mileage, and not break down when you need to get somewhere.

The same thing goes for your body. Maintaining your body requires exercise, movement, and resistance training. You have to keep your body functioning properly, and if you don't use it, you will lose it. Having a regular exercise routine does two things.

It increases the efficiency of your metabolism, which reduces the amount of energy you need to do the same amount of work. Secondly, the more you teach it how to use fat as fuel, the better it becomes and the more readily it will access what you have stored on your body. You will simultaneously become more efficient at using and accessing fuel.

Protein is not a fuel, but it is essential to maintaining the condition of your body. Without protein, nothing you do for fitness and improving performance will work. If carbs and fats are the gas, protein is the oil that keeps everything working.

Want to build muscle? Eat more protein. Want to have better recovery? Eat more protein. Want to get stronger? Eat more protein. Want to sleep better? Eat more protein.

Three things you can do to have more energy

1. Cut out the carbs and get fat-adapted

2. Stop eating extra fat, pre-workout, and other stimulants to give yourself energy.

3. Exercise more with weights and add more variety to your routine.

Your body wants to do what's best for you. If you take care of it, it will take care of you.

Fitness

Fitness is where the rubber meets the road. Improving metabolic function is dependent on building and increasing physical ability. The more you ask your body to do, the better it will process and utilize the resources you make available.

Fitness is increasing your capacity to do work. The more work you can do, the healthier you are.

You don't need to be a gym rat. All you need to do is exercise your freedom through physical activity.

"Optimal physical fitness is my new obsession! I used to view exercise as this thing I "had" to do to offset how much I ate. After all, the more calories I burned, the less I would weigh, right?! I don't remember where I first heard it, but when I was taught to separate exercise from weight loss, my entire paradigm shifted. Fitness is its own standalone goal, separate from weight loss! I never thought to look at it that way before. I never thought to embrace the possibility of becoming a fit person for the sake of my quality of life, NOT just my weight! I've discovered so many of my favorite activities through my quest for fitness. I LOVE to dance, spin, do aerobics, and kickbox. I used to dread lifting weights, but now I LOVE IT! There's nothing like seeing and feeling my strength increase over time." – **Autumn W.**

Fat loss is dead

Ask most people why they workout or watch what they eat, and they'll tell you they want to lose weight, get lean, lose body fat, or slim down.

Many people obsess about what they eat. They spend excessive time doing cardio and looking for ways to increase their fat burn. People spend millions of dollars on supplements that will "speed up" metabolism. Society is preoccupied with losing fat.

THERE'S A BETTER WAY

Wanting to change your body composition is a great goal, and it will improve your health. Here's the thing…Body composition is a ratio of TWO factors.

1. Lean Mass (everything not fat, mostly muscle)
2. Body Fat (just the fat)

Depending on your focus, you can make the change process simple or amazingly complicated and stressful.

I've never met someone over fat who wasn't also under-muscled.

What happens when you focus on fat loss?

To lose fat, you need to have a reductionist mindset. You think in terms of restriction and live in a world of denial.

- Reduction mindset
- Restriction
- Losing
- Moderation
- Passive
- Focused on what you don't do

When you focus on fat loss, that's what you get. The process stops at fat loss. You may see some improvement in health markers, but you haven't improved your physiology. You've just stopped doing things that negatively impact it.

Focusing on fat loss doesn't enable additional function and physical ability, which is the biggest part of improving your quality of life.

What happens when you focus on increasing lean mass?

To increase lean mass, you have to take action and develop a plan to grow and improve physical performance. It's a mindset that adds to instead of taking away.

- Growth mindset
- Satiation
- Growing
- Freedom
- Active
- Focused on what you do

When you focus on gaining lean mass, you improve every aspect of physical and metabolic health, including losing more body fat.

The result is much better, more comprehensive, and rewarding.

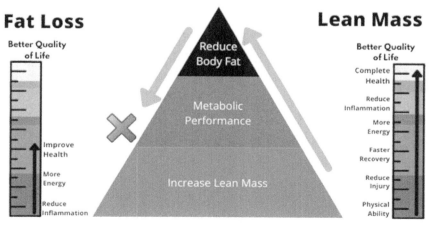

Figure 6 - The Paradigm of Lean Mass

I guarantee your health journey will be much more rewarding, less stressful, and more productive if you focus on the aspect of body composition that improves your quality of life and ability to use your body without limitation.

Step 1. Prioritize protein

- Eat at least 1 gram per pound of lean mass. **Minimum, daily.**
- Eat your protein first at each meal
- If you snack, snack on protein

Step 2. Exercise

- Move weight
- Move well
- Move often

It's not that complicated. Keep it simple. Focus on these basics, and you'll have more long-term success.

You need more muscle

Go to any health coach, personal trainer, or nutritionist, and you won't have any problem finding out how much body fat you should have. The fitness industry is so focused on fat loss that even though many professionals understand the importance of muscle mass, no one has figured out a recommendation for it.

Muscle mass is important for several reasons. It's what allows us to move our bodies. It protects against stress. Muscle improves our metabolic health and helps regulate our hormones. The amount of muscle you have indicates how healthy you are.

"Muscle is perhaps the most important organ system as it relates to combatting our current health crisis, regaining exceptional health, and maximizing physical performance. Muscle is even more important as we age yet is often the most overlooked, even by modern-day medical practices. Muscle is fast becoming the 6th vital sign." - **Dr. Gabrielle Lyon**

How Much does Muscle Matter?

"A substantial proportion of MetS (metabolic syndrome) cases would have been theoretically prevented if prior exposure to low muscle mass and strength were eradicated... Findings indicate that insulin resistance is a central abnormality in the MetS and that muscle mass and strength are strong protective factors independent of insulin resistance and abdominal fat accumulation." – _Inverse associations between muscle mass, strength, and the metabolic syndrome_

"All four outcomes decreased from the lowest quartile to the highest quartile of skeletal muscle index (SMI), the ratio of total skeletal muscle mass (estimated by bioelectrical impedance) to total body weight... Across the full range, higher muscle mass (relative to body size) is associated with better insulin sensitivity and lower risk of PDM

(Diabetes Mellitus)" – *Relative muscle mass is inversely associated with insulin resistance and prediabetes*

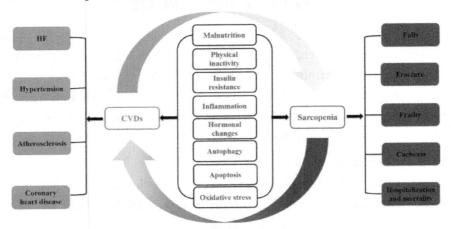

Figure 7 - The Pathogenesis of Sarcopenia

"The pathogenesis of sarcopenia and CVDs (Cardiovascular Disease). Malnutrition, physical inactivity, insulin resistance, inflammation, hormonal changes, autophagy, apoptosis, and oxidative stress are involved in the occurrence of CVDs and sarcopenia. Sarcopenia is closely related to cardiovascular disease, which affects each other's course of the disease. In addition, CVDs aggravates the adverse outcomes of sarcopenia, including falls, fracture, frailty, cachexia, hospitalization, and mortality. At the same time, the prevalence of CVDs in sarcopenia patients is significantly increased, such as HF, hypertension, atherosclerosis, and CHD." – *Relationship Between Sarcopenia and Cardiovascular Diseases in the Elderly: An Overview*

The Fat Standard

Body fat % is the go-to for most people when trying to get healthy. Body fat % is a common metric that aligns with the idea that weight loss is the key to being healthy, except that it's not.

The amount of body fat a person carries is a symptom of an inefficient and improperly managed metabolism. Two main things create conditions of poor metabolic performance and the accumulation of body fat.

1. Not getting enough Nutrient-Dense, Bioavailable, and Satiating food
2. Not doing activities that stimulate muscle growth and improve metabolic performance

Of course, it's a lot more complicated than that, right?

Not really.

Not eating food to optimize your health means you're eating foods that do the opposite. Every bite you take adds to your metabolic dysfunction. Metabolic dysfunction is the source of body fat accumulation.

Guess what else poor nutrition does. It limits your ability to gain and maintain muscle mass. So you end up with more fat AND less muscle.

Living a sedentary lifestyle with little to no movement and stimulation of muscle is a clear path to metabolic problems. Muscle burns fuel, muscle utilizes protein, muscles are the engine that everything you eat supports. If you aren't moving your body, there's nowhere for all that food to go. Nothing is asking for it. The only place your body can put it is in your body fat.

Muscles need activity to grow. Your body responds well to being used, not to sitting still. When you use your muscles, they respond by growing and developing to provide the strength and ability to support what you're asking them to do. If movement is life, you can't have much of one without adequate muscle mass.

The metric of improving health that many people default to is losing body fat. You can see that's not the problem. The issue is most people are under-muscled.

Body Fat % Recommendation Problems

Common body fat recommendations have a couple of issues. First, they are too broad. To "cover the bases," most organizations have provided ranges that allow them to meet the obligation of offering guidance without the risk of being wrong because they were too specific. Secondly, they are based on recorded averages from the current population, not evaluated on a level indicating optimal health.

Common body fat % recommendations look like this.

Body Fat Percentages for Men and Women

Body fat percentage chart for women					
Age	Dangerously low	Excellent	Good	Fair	Poor	Dangerously high
20–29	under 14%	14–16.5%	16.6–19.4%	19.5–22.7%	22.8–27.1%	over 27.2%
30–39	under 14%	14–17.4%	17.5–20.8%	20.9–24.6%	24.7–29.2%	over 29.2%
40–49	under 14%	14–19.8%	19.9–23.8%	23.9–27.6%	27.7–31.9%	over 31.3%
50–59	under 14%	14–22.5%	22.6–27%	27.1–30.4%	30.5–34.5%	over 34.6%
over 60	under 14%	14–23.2%	23.3–27.9%	28–31.3%	31.4–35.4%	over 35.5%

Body fat percentage chart for men					
Age	Dangerously low	Excellent	Good	Fair	Poor	Dangerously high
20–29	under 8%	8–10.5%	10.6–14.8%	14.9–18.6%	18.7–23.1%	over 23.2%
30–39	under 8%	8–14.5%	14.6–18.2%	18.3–21.3%	21.4–24.9%	over 25%
40–49	under 8%	8–17.4%	17.5–20.6%	20.7–23.4%	23.5–26.6%	over 26.7%
50–59	under 8%	8–19.1%	19.2–22.1%	22.2–24.6%	24.7–27.8%	over 27.9%
over 60	under 8%	8–19.7%	19.8–22.6%	22.7–25.2%	25.3–28.4%	over 28.5%

Figure 8 - Body Fat % Averages

There is a giant range based on health, age, and gender. This is bogus. The purpose of making a recommendation is to provide a target for improving health. How is this helpful?

Additionally, I am very passionate about this. Body fat % does not need to increase with age: period, end of story.

When you dig into the data and how health organizations develop these recommendations, you find they are simply percentiles of the general population. Since the general population is obese and unhealthy,

I'm not sure it makes sense to base our body fat % goals on that control group.

Lastly, Body Mass Index (BMI) is still king in the health and medical industry. Many recommendations rely on how body fat is related to BMI and doesn't consider the role muscle mass plays in the equation.

Body Fat % in Context

Optimal health is the goal. That means being fit, NOT being skinny. When I talk about losing body fat, I'm talking about what happens from improving your metabolism and increasing your muscle mass. I am not making a recommendation on how to be skinny.

The following recommendation is an ideal body fat % that indicates optimal health.

Is it the same for everyone? No. Do I think it's a good target for everyone to shoot for? Absolutely.

Body Fat % Recommendations

BF% for Men (All ages)

- 20% or less

BF% for Women (All ages)

- 23% or less

These percentages are a combination of real-world experience and information recorded on populations with a higher average fitness level than the general population. If the goal is optimal health, then targeting averages based on unhealthy people is counter-productive.

Now that we've worked through that, let's dig into the really important stuff.

Fix your muscle. Fix your health.

There are three main components to your body composition.

1. Lean Body Mass (lbs)

2. Body Fat %
3. Skeletal Muscle Mass (lbs)

Lean Body Mass is how much your body weighs minus body fat.

Body Fat % is the amount of body fat in pounds divided by your total weight.

Skeletal Muscle Mass is how much muscle (specifically muscle attached to bone, not organ muscles) you have in pounds.

In the study, "Kwon E, Nah EH, Kim S, Cho S. Relative Lean Body Mass and Waist Circumference for the Identification of Metabolic Syndrome in the Korean General Population 2021 Dec 14", they took data from almost 500,000 people to determine what the cutoff was for the lowest amount of lean mass someone could have before they indicated that they were metabolically unhealthy.

They found that the cut-offs of Relative Lean Body Mass for predicting metabolic syndrome were 74.9% in males and 66.4% in females. That's the same as 25.1% body fat for men and 33.6% for women.

While it's great to know how much lean mass to shoot for, lean mass isn't that easy to manipulate. Luckily, Skeletal Muscle Mass is one very specific component to overall lean body mass that you can change and control very well.

What is Skeletal Muscle Mass Percentage (SMM) %?

Many body composition reports overlook the percentage of skeletal muscle compared to the overall weight, even though it's a more impactful metric than body fat %.

If you weigh 150lbs. and your body fat % is 30%, you have 45lbs of fat on your body. If your skeletal muscle mass is 70lbs, you have a Skeletal Muscle Mass % (SMM%) of 46%.

I found references to 13 different studies that used calculations for SMM% to define the **lower limits** of skeletal muscle mass that indicates sarcopenia (an unhealthy low level of muscle mass) in adults. The overall average across these studies is 31.7% for men and 26.3% for women.

Here's where the fun begins. In the 10+ years, I have been a fitness coach, I have never seen any industry, health, or fitness organization publish a recommendation for SMM%. I have looked, and the only thing I have found is the recorded averages of the general population.

Here is an example from Omron, a large manufacturer of body composition devices.

Skeletal Muscle Percentage

Table 1 - Skeletal Muscle Mass Averages

Male	Female	Classification
5.0 to 32.8%	5.0 to 25.8%	- (Low)
32.9 to 35.97%	25.9 to 37.9%	0 (Normal)
35.8 to 37.3%	28.0 to 29.0%	+ (High)
37.4 to 60%	29.1 to 60%	++ (Very High)

According to this dataset, the average man is about 35% SMM%, and the average woman is 32% SMM%. The average person is only 2.3% higher than the lowest range of defined sarcopenia in men and 5.7% higher for women.

Taking this information into consideration, I looked at people I consider healthy and fit. That is the goal, right?

I looked at data from clients I've worked with, other people in the health and fitness community, and even myself to determine a realistic recommendation that makes sense. I asked two basic questions. 1. Can normal people set it as a health goal? 2. Is it realistic to expect people to get there?

Remember, optimal health is the goal. That means being fit and physically capable. The following recommendation is an ideal SMM% that indicates optimal health.

Is it the same for everyone? No. Do I think it's a good target for everyone to shoot for? Absolutely.

Skeletal Muscle Mass % Recommendations

SMM% For Men (All ages)

- 45% or more

SMM% For Women (All ages)

- 40% or more

You can see this is higher than the Omron "normal" numbers. However, it is lower than the references for "fit" people. My SMM %, for example, is 51%. The median of the fittest individuals in the OMRON data is 49% for men and 45% for women.

In context, these recommendations would mean a 150lbs woman should have 60lbs of SMM, and a 200lbs man should have 90lbs of SMM.

These are solid targets that you can use to help improve your metabolic health. If you change your focus to growing muscle, you will see an overall improvement in your quality of life, physical ability, energy levels, and body fat loss.

Do you know what your body composition is? If you haven't had an opportunity to get a body scan, I highly recommend it. My go-to device is from InBody USA. I trust the accuracy and consistent per-formance of InBody devices so much that I used one for all my members when I owned my CrossFit gym. Many other fitness centers and supple-ment shops have a commercial-grade InBody scale that you can use.

You can also get an at-home device for more convenience. I have one, and I use it regularly.

Getting a good biometric scan provides all the information you need to understand your body composition and where you need to focus. Using this information gives you the power to identify a goal that will help you improve your health. Here are three things you can do to start improving your SMM%

1. Eat more protein. Your body needs it to grow
2. Move more weight. You need to give your body a reason to grow
3. Get more sleep. Your body needs time to grow

That's the basics.

How to build muscle

Obviously, I am a big advocate of building lean mass and improving strength as the foundation for metabolic health, and enhancing your quality of life.

The idea of not focusing on fat loss is foreign to many. Awareness and education of why and how to build lean mass are not discussed or encouraged enough.

It's a better process and mindset to build muscle and get strong as the priority. The process is simple, but it can be challenging to follow through.

When you stop focusing on fat loss, a couple of things change.

You need to stop looking at the scale. Your weight means nothing. Muscle takes up less space than fat. Your weight may not change a single digit as you increase lean mass. You may even gain weight at first.

Shocking, I know. The more important factor in attaining health is the % of fat to lean mass. As you gain muscle, you get healthier. That's what you want. Your clothes will get bigger. You will shrink in size. The scale may not move. That's OK.

Guess what else is going to happen?

You'll likely need to consume more food. Seriously. Most people don't eat enough in general. Many people are very low on how much protein they eat. You'll need to get used to eating a higher quantity of food, particularly protein.

Build muscle mass in 3 easy steps.

Your body only needs three things to start the building process and change everything for you.

1. Adequate protein
2. Adequate physical activity
3. Get more sleep

Protein

Adequate protein starts at 1g per pound of lean mass. If you don't know your lean mass, you can substitute your goal body weight. Your goal weight is generally higher than your lean mass, which isn't bad. When it comes to protein, more is almost always better.

If your lean mass is 150 pounds, you should start targeting 150g of protein per day. The ratio of 1 gram of protein to 1 pound of lean mass is 1:1. Many people I have worked with have a lot of success, around 1.25g-1.5g per pound. As a point of reference, I average 1.5g-1.75g per pound of lean mass.

I want to clarify two things about protein.

First, there is no known upper limit for how much you can utilize at one time. The idea that you can only use 30g of protein per meal is wrong and not historically consistent. Protein is life.

I doubt our ancestors were measuring out 6oz. portions of mammoth after a seven-day fast and hunt.

If 30g of protein were the most you could process at a time, anyone eating three meals a day of 50g per meal would never make any progress because they would be wasting 60g of protein every day. Good thing it doesn't work that way.

Second, the 30g myth was taken from studies that demonstrate the stimulation of Muscle Protein Synthesis (MPS) at 20g to 30g of protein ingested. If you want to gain muscle mass, 30g of protein is a minimum per meal, not a maximum.

When you get your protein is irrelevant. Total daily intake is more impactful on your ability to gain muscle. There is no need to worry about timing your meals around your workouts. Keep it simple and focus on consistency in overall intake.

After a workout, your body increases Muscle Protein Synthesis (MPS) for the next 24hrs to 48hrs. If you are working out 3 to 5 days a week, you are maintaining an elevated state of MPS. Total daily protein intake is all you need to worry about.

Resistance Training

Use this as the starting point and go up as you become more accustomed to the quantity of protein each day.

What exactly is "adequate physical activity? Well, it's moving weight, a lot.

Resistance training is critical in telling your body what to do with all the protein you're going to start taking in. If you're not currently active, you will see an increase in lean mass just off the protein intake. That won't last forever, though. You will need to stimulate muscle growth by moving your body and weight.

Here are some simple guidelines for what weight training should look like for you.

Figuring out how to organize your workout routine is a rabbit hole you could get lost in. The absolute best way to do this correctly and safely is to follow a program and work with someone who can guide you through the process.

The key to weight training is to find a balance between "oh my goodness, that was hard" and "oh crap, I hurt myself". You can do this by keeping your training intensity with weights around a 7-8 out of 10. If you consistently hit this level of challenge, you will see improvement, and you're less likely to get hurt.

You should shoot for at least three days a week, moving weights. The exercises you need to include are squatting, lunging, pulling, pushing, hinging (bending over), twisting, and walking.

People often ask how heavy and how many reps they should do. You should go as heavy as that 7-8 out of 10 lets you go. If you finish a set of 8 reps and feel like you could have done one, maybe two more at the most, you hit the mark. If you feel like it wasn't that hard and you had three or more reps left, you need to go heavier or do more reps.

The ideal rep range for a beginner is 3-12 reps. Within the 3-12 rep range, you can build strength and muscle with a higher degree of safety. You don't need more, and less than three would mean the weight will be heavier than safe.

Sleep

Several things increase your body's affinity to grow muscle, reduce inflammation, and improve recovery when you sleep.

- Cortisol is your body's stress hormone.
- Testosterone is your body's growth hormone.
- Insulin-like Growth Factor (IGF-1) is a major hormone related to lean mass growth.
- Human Growth Hormone (HGH) is a major hormone related to recovery and lean mass growth.

Let's take a look at how sleep affects each of these.

- Cortisol is catabolic (breaking things down) and works on a bell curve, decreasing as you sleep, slowly increasing the closer you get to waking up.
- Testosterone is anabolic (building things up) and works on an opposite bell curve as cortisol.
- IGF-1 increases during sleep.
- IGF-1 improves lean mass
- HGH increases during sleep.
- HGH aids in muscle growth

When you combine these factors with a better understanding of oxidative priority and how the body uses protein, you can see that your body isn't chewing up muscle while you sleep.

In fact, in an environment with adequate fuel (preferably fat) available, muscle mass is maintained. It could increase, on top of the benefits that come with reduced inflammation and better recovery.

If you aren't seeing progress in your training, health, or body composition, take a look at your sleep habits. They are probably keeping you from being your best.

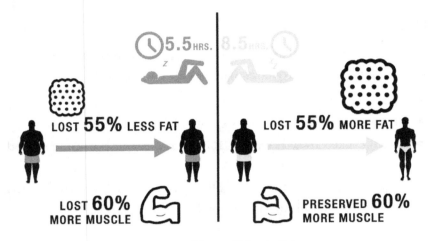

Figure 9 - Sleep and Muscle Gain

These are just some very high-level guidelines that you can use if you're doing this on your own.

I highly recommend following a program and making it easier by letting a professional do the planning and programming part for you.

Building lean mass and completely flipping conventional wisdom on its head is no easy task. It will take some resetting of your belief systems and a daily shift in your mindset. It's 100% worth it.

Eat more protein. Move more weight. Get more sleep.

Why heart rate zone training doesn't work

You need to get in the ZONE. It's all the rage lately. Tons of fancy electronics will tell you when you've entered the FAT BURNING ZONE. You can join fancy gyms with lots of technology, so you know exactly how hard you are working and how long you stay in the "optimal" workout zone.

Wait, what is an "optimal" workout zone?

There are several different ways to work with heart rate-based training zones. If you train at an exertion level of about 65% to 75% of your heart rate, you will be in the best zone to burn fat faster; this is called the "Fat Burning Zone."

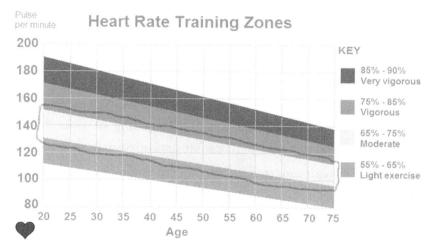

Figure 10 - Heart Rate Training Zones

Technology has allowed us to reliably track when someone's heart rate hit's this zone. Many people consider this the best way to tell if they are working hard enough to see results from their fitness program.

The title of this chapter is "Beware the zone" What is there to beware of? Isn't Heart Rate Training a perfectly valid way to determine the effectiveness of a workout?

How hard someone works isn't the determining factor in the efficacy of their workout.

It certainly plays a role, but what about technique, progressive overload, modality variation, or targeted energy systems?

Heart rate-based training focuses on one aspect of the process and ignores the rest. Doing so eliminates critical aspects of a comprehensive fitness program.

1. Strength training is watered down to something that can keep the heart rate up but doesn't allow for rest intervals or weights heavy enough to develop adequate strength.
2. Variation in movement and exercises are reduced due to the emphasis on high-intensity movement and limitation in the technology to read the effects of certain exercises.
3. Every workout is the same, meaning every workout trains the same energy system and ignores the overall training metabolic flexibility

The goal of improving your fitness is to see verifiable changes in metabolic and physical performance.

I'm not talking about high-level athletes either. People work out for different reasons. The process results in getting stronger, having more endurance and stamina, etc. These are performance-based measures.

Using the heart rate training method to determine performance is like using the tachometer instead of the speedometer to determine how fast you're driving your car.

The goal of a good training program is to increase the amount of work capacity someone has. The underlying premise is that the measurable effect is, in work completed, not the amount of energy used to complete it.

How is the training improving what your body can do?

If it takes a person 5 minutes to walk up 20 flights of stairs, the amount of effort is inconsequential to the amount of time it took. If their training program is working, the next time they climb those stairs, it should only take 4 minutes. That is a measurable improvement.

High intensity without consistency or technique.

The focus is on the intensity at the cost of consistent performance of safe and efficient technique.

Technique first, performed consistently, before increasing intensity is the method for safe, effective, long-term growth and development.

Heart rate-based training starts with intensity for each workout. It's backward to what works best long-term.

Over-training is likely, and burnout can happen when someone is simply "going hard" all the time.

Where's the Coach?

With all this emphasis on keeping the heart rate up, when does coaching happen? Sure there is a trainer to hopefully make sure no one is doing anything egregiously unsafe. How much attention can they pay while focusing on keeping everyone pumped up and working hard?

In a program designed to push you as hard as possible, where is the intake process to find out what you need and what will work best to help you succeed?

There can still be a place in someone's fitness journey for heart rate-based training.

1. It can be super fun, and that can get someone off the couch and into a class. (#winning)
2. Many people who have little to no experience in a gym can benefit from the reduced number of exercises and the program's simplicity.
3. It's easy to understand and grasp the concept of the program. Work hard, get your name into the zone and keep it there.

These programs are great for getting people into their first organized fitness program. There are many success stories of people making fantastic changes by doing these workouts.

While there is a place for all fitness programs, not all programs can maintain someone's fitness journey for years and years.

In many cases, people in heart rate-based programs hit plateaus and cannot break through them until they move on to a more well-rounded and comprehensive program.

At some point in time, most people will need a program based on functional movement where intensity is constantly varied with different movements, exercises, time domains, and energy systems.

What do you do now?

When looking at a program, ask yourself what your goals are and if you think that program will help you get there. Then ask yourself if that program will continue to help you reach the next set of goals after that....and so on.

Intensity and how to make it work for you

You just finished your workout, and you are sweaty, gasping for air, laying on the floor, barely able to get up on your knees, and slowly crawl over to a bench to recover your senses when you hear it from across the room.

"That wasn't so bad."

"Are you freaking serious?!?!" you ask yourself, "That sucked. What's wrong with that guy?!".

There's nothing wrong with that guy. He's just working at a different level of intensity.

"But I thought to get any benefit from exercise. You had to crush yourself every time."

Sure you can, but you don't have to. A good fitness program will have varying intensity levels in each workout.

What is Intensity?

There are three things to consider when talking about intensity.

Absolute Intensity is the work you are doing. If you move 100 pounds, then you just moved 100 pounds. If you ran 1 mile, then you just ran 1 mile. That's it. The measurable work completed is the absolute intensity.

Relative Intensity is the % of the effort required to complete the work based on an individual's fitness level. If the most you can move is 200 pounds and you move 100 pounds, your relative intensity is 50%. If Nancy can move 400 pounds and she moves 100 pounds, then her relative intensity is 25%.

The focus of any fitness program should be to increase your ability in both Absolute and Relative Intensity.

The Rate of Perceived Exertion (RPE) is the one that gets people all messed up, and this is where we're going to focus our discussion. RPE is 100% based on how hard a person *feels* they are working.

When most people talk about intensity in a workout, they're talking about RPE. "That workout crushed me!" It's a subjective observation about how much energy they feel they put into the work. It's the same as when someone says, "Oh, that wasn't so bad."

These two points of view can and often do exist simultaneously. They're related

When you first start a new fitness routine, everything seems hard. You aren't worried about how much weight you're using or how fast you do the work. You're just worried about getting through the workout. You want to perform the movements safely and correctly. That's where your focus is (and should be).

Your Absolute and Relative Intensities are low. Your RPE is high. Everything seems hard.

After a while, you get more comfortable with the movements, and you sense that you can go faster or use a heavier weight. Your Absolute and Relative Intensities are increasing. As this increases, your RPE decreases. The work "feels" easier even though you may be doing more measurable work.

The key is to find a way to increase your RPE again. Increasing the level of effort is the key to improving your overall fitness.

Here's the kicker

How do you know when this happens and what to do about it? If the work feels easier, then you should make it harder right? Isn't that what getting better is all about?

The amount of work you can do as you get more in shape should increase. How hard it feels to do that work should stay the same.

I can't count how often I've heard a relatively new person tell me that the workouts aren't challenging. "I'm getting bored. The workouts aren't hard enough."

My response…. "Then make it harder."

What's written in the program does not determine how hard you work or the effort you put into it. If you feel like the workouts are easy, it's because you're getting better!

Now go make it hard again!

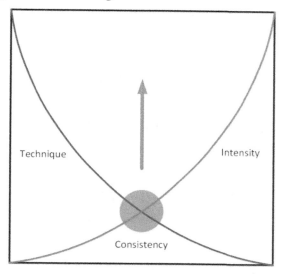

Figure 11 - Fitness Level Progression

If your fitness program is working, you will and should reach a period where things seem easier than they did before. You will know this by how you feel. If you are tracking your performance, you'll know it by looking at the evidence in the numbers.

If you aren't tracking your performance, then it's going to be very hard to know when it's time to increase your RPE through additional Relative Intensity in your workouts.

You won't know how fast you did this workout last time, so you can try and go faster this time. You won't know what weight you used last time, so you can use a heavier weight this time.

Anyone who is not tracking their performance is not serious about improving their health. It's the most important part of the process.

Getting better in three easy steps

Three things affect or create an intensity that you can use to improve your fitness and get a more intense feeling out of your workouts.

Technique – Focus on getting better at executing a movement. The better you perform a movement, the more you'll get out of it.

Weight – Lifting or moving more weight than before is a hallmark for improving your fitness. How can you expect gains if you always pick up the same dumbbell?

Time – The speed at which you move is a sure-fire way to get more intensity into your workouts. How much more speed? Only your past performance can tell you that.

Past performance is the map that will guide you to improved health and fitness.

Just the beginning

Here's the cool part of the whole process.

Intensity works two ways! You can increase it or decrease it as needed.

Because fitness is a personal journey, each person has different needs. While one person may be looking for more intensity, another may need less.

Someone new to fitness needs less intensity as their body and central nervous system grow into the new routine. A person who just had back surgery needs a level of intensity that their newly repaired body can handle without breaking again.

Whatever fitness program you choose, make sure it has coaching and flexibility to allow for whatever level of intensity YOU need. There is no "one size fits all" in fitness. Your story and goals are different. Your training should be too.

Take your time

There are a million workout plans out there. All of them can be intimidating to someone who isn't familiar with exercise, fitness terminology or just hasn't spent a lot of time in a gym environment. Even if you used to work out years ago, there's a natural apprehension to getting started doing physical exercise again.

We've all been there. I have to deal with the mental game, even if I just take a week off. It's normal.

Here's the key to getting started, staying motivated, not getting hurt, and being successful in building a lifestyle of fitness.

TAKE YOUR TIME. That's it. It's that simple.

Understand where you are and approach the activity appropriately.

DO

- Focus on learning the exercises with little to no weight
- Spend more time in the warm-up and cool-down portion of the workouts
- Ask your coach or trainer for feedback.
- Be ok with stopping if you feel like it's too much
- Focus less on speed or how much you finish
- Pay attention to how you feel after your workout
- Get as much sleep as possible
- Eat more protein
- Make sure you are getting a variety of activities

DON'T

- Try and go heavy or fast before you're ready
- Workout every day
- Do the same thing all the time

- Think you're doing something correctly without getting someone to evaluate you
- Rush through the warm-up or cool-down

A good workout program has options for you to modify movements to fit your experience, equipment, or physical ability. A good program provides the opportunity to adjust how much of the workout you do on any given day. It's very common for people to build up to doing the whole daily workout over time if the program supports that.

Bottom line.... The only person you have to prove anything to is yourself. No one else is putting any pressure on you. Don't put too much on yourself. Take your time. Do what makes sense for where you are until you can do more.

There may even be times when you just need to take a day and rest your mind. Do something to destress, or only do part of the workout. That's perfectly fine. The most important thing is to stay in a routine and do what's best for you.

If you're patient, you'll do stuff you never thought possible. You'll do it safely and faster than expected.

Finding a fitness program

If there's one thing I hope you've picked up to this point, it's that fitness is not about looks. It's about improving your body's ability to do things. Your nutrition and fitness lifestyle affect three main areas of your physical ability.

When you start a fitness program, these are the things you should keep an eye out for. If what you're doing doesn't have these components, it may work for a while, but I promise you will stall until you include each one.

Movement, Metabolism, and the Components of Fitness

Your body is designed to move. You cannot live without movement. How well you move determines your independence and self-sufficiency. If you move well, you will have more physical freedom. You need to be able to do these seven functional movements.

These are the basics. There are thousands of variations and levels of complexity and intensity. If you're just starting, keep it simple.

1. Squat - Sitting down and standing up
2. Lunge - Balance and coordination, walking up stairs
3. Hinge - Using your hips to bend, not your back
4. Push - Moving weight away from your body
5. Pull - Moving weight towards your body
6. Carry/Walk - Controlling weight and direction under stress
7. Twist - Maintaining spine support and stabilization

If you are moving your body, you'll need to improve how your body uses energy and what conditions your body can do work. Your metabolic capacity is your engine and how hard you can make your body go.

There are three different ways your body uses fuel. The kind of work and how long you are doing it determines the fuel used.

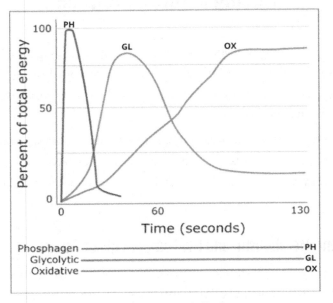

Figure 12- 3 Metabolic Pathways

When you perform a very short burst high-intensity effort like lifting a heavy weight one time, you're using the Phosphagen/ATP Pathway. The ATP Pathway uses energy stored in the cells to provide the movement necessary to generate the force and perform the movement

Slightly longer work periods where glycogen stored in the muscle is the primary energy source is called the Glycolytic Pathway. You use the Glycolytic Pathway in sprints and High-Intensity Interval Training (HIIT).

The way your body supplies fuel for longer endurance work like running, swimming, or biking is the Oxidative Pathway. It mainly uses fat and oxygen to provide energy.

To optimize your nutrition and metabolic capacity, you need to include each of these pathways in your fitness routine.

Combining the 7 Essential Movements and the 3 Metabolic Pathways gives you a comprehensive change in your physiology and nervous system. You improve how your physical hardware and internal circuitry work together.

This is where the 10 Components of Fitness impact your everyday life.

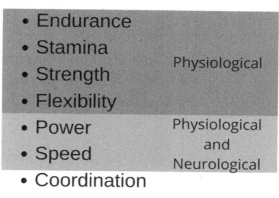

Figure 13 - 10 Components of Fitness

Your ability to perform in each component indicates your overall health and quality of life. These are the things you should look for when you are getting started.

"Constantly Varied, Functional Movement, Performed at High Intensity." This is the definition that Greg Glassman, the creator of CrossFit, gives for that program. It is a perfect summation of everything I just went through.

You need variety, different levels of intensity, mental and skill development, and simple, easily performed but challenging exercises.

Your life has a lot of different demands on it, and stress comes in many forms. Your fitness has to be able to handle all of it.

Meet you where you are.

A good fitness program includes all of this, and it has the flexibility and adaptability to meet you where you are. A good program builds scaling and modifications into the culture and workout design.

A program might not be right for you if there are no options for your current physical ability, environment, available equipment, etc.

Specific Adaptation to Imposed Demand

Remember, your body will only adapt to the level you require it. If you want to be live a physically unrestricted life, you need to put the demands of that life into your everyday routine.

How to get the most out of your workouts

Now that you know what you're looking for, what are some things you can do to get the most out of your program?

You want to make progress quickly, but make sure you stay safe. You probably have a busy schedule, so time management is a consideration. Here are four things you can do to optimize your time doing fitness activities and boost your progress.

Always do the Warm-up. Warm-ups have two main functions. First, they prepare your body for the level of intensity you are about to experience. Without a good warm-up, the risk of injury during your workout greatly increases.

Secondly, warm-ups put your body in a position to benefit from the stimulus you apply in the workout. If you jump right into a workout without a good warm-up, your body isn't ready, and it spends a good part of the workout just acclimating to the new level of effort. You get less blood flow, decreased range of motion, lower muscle fiber engagement, and a loss of overall benefit from the workout.

Understand and apply transferability in movement. Everything we do is built on patterns of movement. Our joints and muscles can only do so many things. Seven basic movements make up the foundation of everything we do. Once you understand how to perform one aspect of a movement, learn to apply that to other exercises.

Core engagement is the same no matter what exercise you're doing. If you can learn how to do it when you're doing a plank, it should improve your squat. The mechanics of a lunge, a squat, and a deadlift have similar patterns. When you train one of them, you can transfer that skill to the others.

Understanding how movement patterns transfer from one exercise to another will save you time, help you connect with your body, and improve your skill across the board very quickly.

Move in as great a range of motion as possible. Range of motion is one of the biggest hacks to improve your training results. Focusing on proper technique and range of motion helps you engage more muscle fibers, build stability, and increase energy expenditure.

Your muscles come in different sizes. If you move your joints only half of the distance they can move, you only engage the short to medium length muscles and leave a good portion of muscle fiber inactivated. This common mistake has a double effect of 1. limiting the potential growth of overall muscle mass and 2. compromising strength and stability when putting yourself in an untrained position.

If you never train your overhead press with full extension of your arms, you never prepare your shoulders for the stress to stabilize that position. If something happens in real life that requires you to reach overhead quickly to stop something or lift something, you will likely injure yourself.

The more muscle you activate when you workout, the more energy you require. One way to get the most metabolic benefit from exercise is to make sure you're using as much muscle as possible.

Range of motion is one way to engage and improve strength and stability. Increasing the amount of time moving weight is another one. Time under tension is a concept applied to exerting control and being deliberate in the execution of an exercise.

Increase time under tension. Time under tension means that your muscles are engaged for longer within each rep. The individual reps add up to greater overall exposure to the weight being moved, so the effect on the muscle is greater.

Increasing your time under tension will also develop an improved mind-muscle connection, coordination, and accuracy in movement.

These are components of fitness that will add to your training effect without you having to do specific, extra training.

If you consistently apply these concepts to your fitness routine, you will see a dramatic improvement in not only your fitness but in how well you move, your energy levels, speed of recovery, and overall quality of life.

How to work around an injury

Whether you start your fitness journey with an existing injury or something happens to you along the way, you need to have a process for working through it.

The first thing to understand is that having an injury doesn't mean you can't do anything. Yes, some things can happen where you need to limit all activity. This kind of injury is rare and what I'm addressing here is the kind of injury that causes a disruption to your routine or method but doesn't mean you have to stop everything.

Remember that even though you want to work on your fitness, healing and recovery from the injury are the priority. Never compromise the healing progress or your safety for a workout.

Here are seven things you can do to keep your fitness progress moving forward, even if you get hurt.

Work with a professional and ask for help finding an alternative. You probably aren't trained as a Physical Therapist or have experience rehabilitating an injury. I recommend getting some help and hands-on guidance from a medical professional.

Focus on what you can do. Do not fall into the victim trap. If you can stay focused on the other areas you can still improve, you will develop a deeper appreciation for your body and pride in yourself. There are 20 different components of fitness that are just the foundation for areas you can work. The combinations are endless.

Play around and get curious about how your body works. You have an opportunity to do things you may have never thought about before. Experiment with new types of exercise, movement, and activities. You may find a new passion or experience something that excites you about what your body can do.

Limit the range of motion. Some injuries may allow limited movement. In these cases, it's often a good idea to use what range you have under very controlled intensity.

Reduce the weight or intensity of the movement. This one should go without saying. Always work within safe levels of intensity. Do not compromise your recovery just to feel good about a workout. It's better to stop in the middle of a workout than push through and extend your recovery or make an injury worse.

Avoid the injured area altogether. Your training may need a complete overhaul for a while. You may have to avoid a whole section of your body. That means you need to mentally prepare for lower training volume and focus on the other six things on this list.

Use an aid or equipment to compensate. Many different devices can help you continue a fitness routine while rehabilitating an injury. Finding out what can work for your situation is one of the things a fitness or medical professional can help you figure out. They'll even show you how to use it properly.

Lastly, injuries often happen due to improper technique or too much intensity. Getting hurt is a perfect time to learn how to prevent the injury from happening again. Don't waste your time feeling bad for yourself. Stay positive, and get to work!

For the endurance enthusiasts

If you know anyone who runs a lot or rides bikes for long distances, you know how passionate they are about their sport. If you are an endurance athlete, I envy your enjoyment of the sport. Not many people could do what you do and love it.

Over the years, I have trained many endurance athletes. When I implemented a program that introduced these three things, every athlete saw improvements in endurance and speed.

Increase the variation of training. Endurance sports are repetitive, and overuse is the most common reason for decreased performance and injury in endurance athletes. Repeatedly doing the same movements leads to a maximum training effect for that movement pattern. Once that movement pattern, muscles, tendons, and central nervous system have been trained, where else is there to go?

Variation in your training program is the best way to increase the development of your body without overworking the systems you need to be at their best. You can and need to get better by practicing your sport, to a point. Diminishing returns can ruin the positive effect of your training. Effective training allows for offloading the focus while enhancing the systems being developed.

Take some time and work on your cardiovascular endurance by getting on a rowing machine instead of running or biking. It works the same metabolic systems but saves the movement pattern from getting overworked.

Instead of going on that bike ride today, go throw weight on your shoulders and climb a few hills. Build some muscle mass, you won't have to work so hard, and it will help you last longer on your rides.

Train more strength. Severely misunderstood, strength training is NOT something that will slow you down as an endurance athlete. I'm not talking about trying to become a bodybuilder.

I'm talking about strength training for a couple of specific purposes.

- It allows the muscles to use less energy while they work. Stronger muscles don't work as hard as weaker muscles. It's that simple.
- More muscle mass helps your body reduce the effect of repetitive movement in your joints. With a higher number of muscles fibers to handle the stress of movement, your ligaments and tendons have to deal with less.

Run or bike longer with less energy used and less damage to your body throughout the activity.

Add a consistent mobility routine. Lack of mobility in endurance athletes is a huge problem. It goes beyond the sports performance realm and negatively affects their quality of life.

Mobility combines flexibility, range of motion, and motor strength. It is the ability to put your body into the positions needed to move safely, every time, under stress.

Signs of poor mobility can be lower back pain, hip misalignment, sore knees, painful shoulders, and many others. Your performance as an athlete will suffer if you cannot put your body into good positions. Sure, you may be able to run, bike, and swim, but if every part of your body isn't moving properly when you do it, how much are you leaving on the table?

Poor mobility also points to unhealthy muscles. Tight, sore muscles do not operate efficiently. It's like tying your arms to the side of your body, then trying to jump rope. It just doesn't work.

Bonus: Increase your recovery time and or frequency – FACT: Performance increases only happen during rest periods. You cannot get better unless you rest. It's science, don't fight it. Increasing the amount you rest can work miracles in how fast you get better at your chosen sport. More on that here:

Additionally, the common injuries among endurance athletes are repetitive use injuries like tendonitis, strains, shin splints, plantar fasciitis, etc. Don't let these happen to you.

The body is complex. It is a machine that requires ALL of its parts to be in working order if you want it to perform at its best. Don't spend all your time on one part of the fitness puzzle. Put the whole picture together, and you will improve your specific activity without compromising the rest of your health.

We need strong women

Over the years, I have worked with hundreds of women. You've read my Mom's story. I am emotionally invested in this topic. This book is for everyone. This chapter is for any woman who isn't sure what they can or should be doing to improve their health.

I'm concerned about the alarming number of women who identify or evaluate their fitness based on how they look. Many women I talk to have issues with their appearance that quite literally affects their health, and they don't even know it.

Many women think that being skinny equals being fit. If I had a nickel for every time I've heard "*I don't want to get too bulky.*" or "*I just want to get toned.*", I'd be a rich man.

This mindset is a problem for a couple of reasons.

First and foremost, basing a fitness program on how you think you're going to look is a recipe for failure. Looks are subjective, and in your own eyes, you will never look as good as you want to. If you're basing your looks on how other people see you, you will always be chasing someone else's opinion, which is a dangerous road to go down.

Without defined performance measures, it is much harder to stay consistent and know whether a program is working for you or not. There must be an objective way to determine success.

Strong women don't need affirmation from others, and they know that being fit is about what you can do, the amount of stress your body can handle, and how free you are to do the things you want to do.

If you are fit, then you will look like you're fit.

This fear is based on the idea that muscle is bad. Thinking that muscle is to be avoided is dangerous. Muscle promotes bone density, burns fat, manages hormones, provides safety in movement, and enables the body to perform activities.

Women who don't train with heavy weights are weaker, more prone to injury, at risk for osteoporosis, have higher body fat, and are less active.

Women need muscle. If you weigh 135 pounds and have 35% body fat, you are obese. If you weigh 135 pounds and have 23% body fat, you're probably in pretty good shape with a good amount of muscle. (See how I'm using objective data, based on science, not looks).

This aversion to muscles weakens women physically and perpetuates the perception that women should be small and weak. **It is unacceptable**.

If you are looking for a fitness program, stop using your looks as a barrier to getting started. The mindset that evaluates looks first misses true health and fitness opportunities. It forces you into an inferior program with fewer real-life benefits and keeps you weak and superficial.

There is nothing wrong with a strong woman. There is everything RIGHT with a strong woman.

Women experience stressful situations just like men. Why should they be weak? If more women viewed their fitness as a tool to empower themselves and create a new level of freedom, the world would be a better place.

We need strong women.

Nutrition

In this section, I want to walk you through why nutrition is important. More importantly, I want you to understand why it must be combined with fitness. You need both.

My approach to nutrition is simple. There is an optimal way for humans to eat.

I provide information that may surprise you and contradict things you thought you knew. I also provide some practical tools and information to help you implement these concepts to work for your specific situation.

"During my mid-twenties to mid-thirties, my health and weight fluctuated. I gained nearly fifty pounds, developed pre-diabetes, suffered from depression, and fell into a dangerous lifestyle of alcohol and recreational drug abuse. When I hit 40, I knew enough was enough and was ready to transform myself from the man I was to the man I wanted to be. So I embarked on a path of sobriety that has led to positive lifestyle adjustments that affect my diet and fitness.

Nutrition plays a big role in my life. I tried the whole vegetarian thing for several years, and in the beginning, it was great. However, I began to feel like crap, and after a while, I ditched veggies and carbs for intermittent fasting and Keto. Within two weeks, I noticed a big difference in my overall health. I was more alert had better focus, but I still had occasional bloating. That all changed when I switched to eating Carnivore about a year and a half ago. So between that and intermitted fasting, I'm rocking and rolling." **– Glenn P.**

Nutrition is only half the solution

You've spent the last several years feeling bad. You're sick, tired, and frustrated. You finally have had enough and start to change your eating habits. It takes time, but you start to see improvement. Your digestion issues get better. You have more energy. The chronic issues or conditions you were dealing with go away. You feel amazing!!

You finally have your life back!

Improving your nutrition fixes many health issues resulting from poor lifestyle habits. Fixing health problems with nutrition may lead you to believe there is no need for a fitness routine to gain health. Technically this conclusion is correct, sort of.

It depends on how you define "health". Let's set a baseline.

What is the natural state of the human body?

The human body's natural state is not one of chronic inflammation and stress. Unfortunately, this is a state far too many people are in. Changing your nutrition habits will bring you closer to where your body wants to be.

What you eat will help you reduce the stress and extra work that your body is dealing with on the inside.

How do I know if I have excess internal stress? Do you have any of these issues or something similar?

- Insulin resistance
- Obesity
- Hypertension
- IBS
- Crohns
- Eczema
- Psoriasis

- Acne
- Hashimoto's
- Polycystic Ovarian Syndrome (PCOS)
- Colitis
- Cardiovascular disease
- And on, and on, and on…

If your body is functioning without chronic stress and inflammation, you are healthy.

If normal function and healthy are the same, where are you right now?

Any state other than healthy is below the baseline of function for the human body. Improving your health means working to get back to the basic level where your body wants to be.

Think about that…— the basic level of function.

Getting there is a huge accomplishment. It's a phenomenal achievement to look in a mirror and say, "I'm healthy again!". The impact on your life is very real, and the freedom you gain from attaining health is life-altering.

But it's limited.

Nutrition habits will get you to baseline. The result is the equivalent of fixing a car to run fine in a garage, quick trips to the grocery store, or teaching your kid how to drive. It works well enough, but don't push it. If you do, it will break.

Healthy nutrition habits get your body to function well in the **absence of internal stress**. It is the process of removing stress from your body.

Having a well-rounded fitness routine improves your body's ability to perform in any situation, even in the **presence of external stress**.

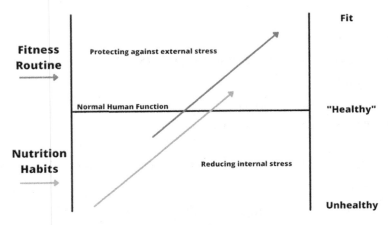

Figure 14 - Fitness and Nutrition Overlap Health

You do not live in a world without external pressures, stress, physical needs, and requirements. Without including a process for preparing your body to perform efficiently, sustainably, and effectively, you don't stand a chance to maintain any health, you may have gained by changing your nutrition for very long.

What do you need to handle stress, perform physical activity, and build a sustainable, well-functioning physiology?

- Efficient metabolic function
- Muscle mass
- Mental toughness
- Strength
- Endurance
- Stamina
- Power
- Flexibility
- Stability
- Balance
- Coordination
- Accuracy
- Agility

Nutrition can teach your body how to use fuel properly. Fitness makes it more efficient.

Nutrition can give your body the material to build lean mass and muscle. Fitness does the building.

Nutrition cannot improve any components of fitness that directly impact your body's ability to do work and perform under pressure.

Nutrition cannot improve your ability to move your body safely without the risk of injury.

Nutrition cannot give you confidence in your physical capability or increase physical freedom.

I hope this helps you understand why it's important to include fitness in your routine. If you don't, you miss out on everything you need to help you thrive for many years and the freedom and enjoyment of being physically fit.

Eating less and still getting fat

Calories in calories out.

Did you know that not every calorie is equal?

As a general rule, you can use caloric intake to reduce your weight and even improve your health.

But it only goes so far. Reducing your calories for a long-term period can have serious side effects.

There's the problem with the "calories in calories out" model. It doesn't affect any positive long-term metabolic changes.

When you use the amount of food you eat as the controlling factor for fat loss and health, you constantly change your body's ability to function efficiently.

Reducing calories means reducing nutrients. Fats, protein, carbs, and all the vitamins and minerals your body needs will be low at times, then high at times. The constant back and forth can wreak havoc on your system.

If you go on a long-term calorie reduction, you will see overall weight loss at the expense of muscle loss. Remember, the less muscle you have, the less healthy you are. Muscle mass is super important to your overall health.

The more muscle you have, the less risk you are at having metabolic syndrome, cardiovascular disease, diabetes, osteoporosis, and sarcopenia.

Three major things happen on a calorie-restricted diet. Your body has fewer nutrients and is less able to function. Your metabolic performance decreases (inefficient metabolism)

Your body gets fewer nutrients and is less able to function. Your metabolic performance decreases, which reduces the amount of energy it uses. Fewer tools and resources to work with means less work gets done. It's not slower fuel burning. It's less functionality. Your body is literally on a work stoppage.

When you diet using a caloric deficit, you reduce the overall nutrient density of your food. Even though you've reduced your calories, the reduction in nutrients and metabolic activity puts you in a net negative of fuel utilization. When nutrient density goes down, caloric density goes up. Essentially the ratio of calories to function is put out of balance, and your body will have extra fuel it can't use. You will get to a point where you lose muscle and gain body fat.

When your body lacks nutrients, it has to get them from somewhere. You lose lean mass or have hormone dysfunction in an extended caloric deficit because your body will catabolize itself to keep you alive. Caloric deficit dieting is by definition a form of starvation. Calcium gets pulled from bones, amino acids from muscle, and other nutrients from wherever your body can get them.

The results of extended caloric restriction include.

- Fatigue
- Poor sleep
- Hair loss
- Fat gain
- Poor insulin management
- Weight doesn't change
- Irritability

This chapter is Titled "Eating less and still getting fat", what if I told you, you could eat more and still get skinny???

You can! Improve your metabolic function and improve your fat loss and overall health. It is impossible to improve metabolic function and starve your body of nutrients at the same time.

The idea of caloric restriction isn't completely wrong. It has its roots in a very solid concept, but how the human body functions and how you live your life make it work differently in reality.

Eat more and get skinny

I did a little experiment a while ago. I chowed down like never before, and I lost body fat. I had been eating 1800 to 1900 calories per day to try and lose weight. I changed it up and started eating an average of 2600 calories per day, and all I did was lose body fat. I increased the amount of food I was eating by 700 - 800 calories. I still lost body fat!!

I would have added body fat if I had eaten that amount of food on my old, carb-focused diet. My activity level hadn't changed. I was just eating more and losing body fat. How does that happen???

Fat is magic! Not really, but close.

Mitochondria

These little guys are the workhorses of our metabolism. The more you have and the better they work, the less stress your body has to deal with, and the more energy you can utilize throughout the day.

When you say you are "speeding up" your metabolism, you're saying that you are optimizing your mitochondrial production and performance to increase your body's ability to burn fuel.

Guess what the best way is to help those mitochondria function, cutting out the carbs and adding in more fat.

"See, mitochondria burn fatty acids cleaner than they burn carbohydrates. Generating ATP via fats/ketones produces fewer free radicals, because it's more efficient, whereas generating ATP via carbs produces more" – Excerpt from https://www.marksdailyapple.com/managing-your-mitochondria/

Eating more fat improves your metabolic performance. That explains why I can eat more than before and still lose fat. I'm burning more than I was before with an inefficient metabolism.

Brown Fat

There are two types of body fat. White Fat and Brown Fat. White Fat stores energy and Brown Fat burns energy. Guess what is inside Brown Fat that makes it burn energy.

Mitochondria!

Brown Fat burns energy for fun. It's almost like its sole job is to regulate our body fat like a release valve. All it does is burn fat.

Guess how you increase the amount of brown fat in your body while reducing white fat?

Eat fewer carbs and burn more fat. Being fat-adapted, where the body is relying on ketones for fuel, increases metabolic rate by increasing the amount of brown fat and mitochondria in your body.

Protein makes a difference

The other thing I did during this experiment, besides cutting out the carbs, was to increase my protein intake. I was eating over 2x my lean mass by pounds in grams of protein.

Keep this information in mind as you get further into nutrition and learn how food works in your body. For now, remember, protein is not a fuel. Your body is protein storage. It's nearly impossible to overeat protein.

Protein does not turn to fat in your body.

Summary

Eating a very low carb/zero carb diet puts us in a position to:

- Remove carbs and become fat-adapted
- Providing fat as fuel for mitochondria improves fuel utilization
- Reduces oxidative stress and free-radicals
- Allows for enhanced body fat loss regardless of caloric intake

Also, prioritizing protein is a great way to improve your body composition without worrying about overeating.

Sign me up!!

How to do caloric deficit correctly

Let's recap what your metabolism is and why it matters in the context of calories.

First, your metabolism is not how fast your body burns fuel.

No matter how much cardio you do or how many calories you think you burn during a workout, you aren't doing anything that helps long-term success.

The idea of being in a deficit is a simple equation. If your body burns X, eat X − (some amount), and lose weight.

Losing weight and reducing body fat are two very different things. Focusing on weight loss messes people up and probably has had you on yo-yo diets or off again on again cycles of diet and exercise.

Your metabolism is the total of what your body does every day to keep you alive. It is all your biological, physiological, and neurological systems and mechanisms.

The amount of fuel you consume or burn off is just one piece of the puzzle.

Think about this for a minute. If Calories In, Calories Out worked, why are an increasing number of people sick with metabolic syndrome year after year after year? Around 70% of the US population has some form of metabolic syndrome!

The idea of being "in a deficit" is antique, oversimplified, and needs to end.

A good body recomposition plan aims to improve metabolic function by maintaining nutrient density and supporting the utilization of stored fuel over external fuel intake.

1. Improve metabolic function
2. Reduce fuel consumption

3.   Burn body fat

How do you reduce fuel consumption without starving yourself and realizing all the problems with a caloric deficit I just mentioned?

Not everything you eat is fuel.

What you eat is broken up into two basic components: Fuel Calories and Functional Calories. Fuel calories (fat and carbs) provide **energy** for the body to function. Functional calories (protein) provide **resources** that enable the body to function. These are two very different things.

A good calorie deficit plan focuses on maintaining functional calories while reducing fuel calories. Prioritizing protein is essential to staying healthy.

Muscle mass drives your metabolism. A good plan will do everything it can to support the maintenance and growth of muscle tissue. That means protein and resistance training is a priority.

Body composition is more effective than bodyweight at tracking your progress.

Your Base Metabolic Rate (BMR) indicates how efficient your metabolism is. If you follow a good body recomposition plan, you should maintain or even increase your BMR. If your BMR is dropping as you progress, that's a good sign you aren't prioritizing protein or doing the physical work needed to stimulate muscle growth.

Your muscle mass should not be dropping. It may even go up. Most body composition scales have a Lean Body Mass (LBM) or Skeletal Muscle Mass (SMM) reading they provide. Use these to track your progress.

When you reduce fuel calories, your body will start to use what's stored. Body fat will become a major source of energy for you. The amount of fuel calories you reduce doesn't need to be drastic.

The more you reduce at once, the less time your body has to adapt to the change. If you make big changes and aren't allowing yourself to adapt, you will see stalls, drops in energy levels, poor digestion, bad sleep, etc.

Fuel Calorie reduction pointers

1. Drop around 50-100 calories per week
2. If you start seeing a drop in body fat, stay there for a bit. If you lose a pound or two of body fat after a week, keep those calories at that level until you don't see any more loss. Cutting more doesn't always mean losing more. Be patient. Play the long game.
3. Don't declare a stall in less than 4-6 weeks
4. Most people don't need to be at less than 70g of fat per day. If you get there and don't see changes, the problem isn't your fuel intake.
   a. You need more protein
   b. You need to start some exercise
   c. You need more sleep
   d. You need to reduce stress
   e. …something else is going on. Get professional help.
5. You don't need to stay in a deficit forever. Some people can do it for a long time. Others need to cycle their fuel intake up and down based on how they feel. One thing is certain. Your health is always more important than how you think you look. Never sacrifice your health.

BIG NOTE: Fuel calorie reduction is a part of improving your metabolism and health. I put this information here because it's important. Do not take the few lines of information about fat loss and turn them into a focus for tracking your progress. Getting better at burning body fat is part of the process. It's not all there is.

How you function is always better to focus on than anything else. Please remember that.

Keto and alcohol don't mix

I am a bourbon guy. I love trying new bourbons, and I have several that I enjoy drinking. I used to have one glass of bourbon 3 to 4 nights a week. In the past, I've had issues limiting myself to drinking one Manhattan a night.

I still enjoy a good Blanton's or Woodford Double Oaked occasionally. I have, however, cut back significantly since I realized the effects it had on my body and health.

A while ago, I went on a 21-day nutrition challenge and didn't drink for three weeks. It wasn't that hard to do, but the results were eye-opening.

- I slept like a rock on a log. Every night I had the best sleep ever.
- I didn't feel as sore from workouts
- I lost 9lbs. **of fat** in 3 weeks! Not total weight, JUST FAT

After these results, I did a little more digging to determine why these things happened. I had a pretty good diet already before I did the challenge. The only change I made was the reduction of alcohol I drank each week.

Here's what I learned.

Oxidative Priority

Alcohol hijacks your metabolism. It stops the body from using fat for fuel, increases inflammation in pretty much every system in your body, and causes dehydration. These things lead to weight gain, slower muscular recovery, poor sleep quality, and an overall reduction in your ability to use fuel (body fat or ketones) and perform well.

Alcohol turns into Acetate. By itself, Acetate is not a harmful substance. It's also a by-product of Ketogenesis. Acetate from alcohol metabolism is a case of too much of a good thing. Acetate forces itself into the front of the metabolic fuel line and won't let your body burn anything else for fuel.— No more body fat burning for you.

Note: Alcohol also breaks down into Acetaldehyde which is highly toxic and causes damage to the body on a cellular and genomic level.

Hormones

Alcohol decreases hormones that build muscle tissue and increases hormones that break muscle tissue down. If you are trying to gain lean mass by eating more protein and increasing the amount of resistance training you do, alcohol is working against you.

The two main hormones you need to build muscle are Insulin-like Growth Factor (IGF-1) and Testosterone. Alcohol suppresses both.

Do you know what else alcohol does? It raises cortisol. Cortisol is your body's primary stress hormone. It's associated with chronic inflammation and all the various issues that come with it.

Lastly, alcohol may inhibit your body's ability to break down estrogen. You end up with more estrogen in your system while slowing down testosterone production.

Sleep

Alcohol tricks the brain into falling asleep fast then keeps poking it all night, so you wake up more tired. Alcohol disrupts REM sleep. So even if you think it helps you sleep, the sleep you're getting is of poor quality and not as beneficial to your progress. If you're falling asleep with alcohol in your system, any anabolic benefit you're getting is negated because IGF-1 and testosterone are suppressed.

Don't get me wrong. I'm not saying you should cut out alcohol altogether. I suggest you evaluate your consumption and see for yourself what effect making some changes could have on how your fitness and health improve.

I haven't even mentioned the caloric, sensitivity, or ingredient issues involved with alcoholic beverages, beers, mixed drinks, etc. Everything you put into your body plays a role in your health. Many people discount the importance alcohol can have.

Don't.

Ketogenic diet getting started guide

The Ketogenic Diet has been an effective tool for many years to help people with all sorts of issues heal themselves and live better lives.

A ketogenic, whole food and animal-based diet has helped many people heal numerous diseases and chronic illnesses. The benefits to metabolic health are the most impressive aspects of the diet.

How does the ketogenic diet do all this and help you lose body fat, gain muscle, and make you feel more energized?

Some things we know.

- Carbohydrates are used for fuel before body fat. If you're putting carbs into your system, losing body fat will always be challenging.
- Most processed foods are carbs. Think about that for a minute. Now think about the first item on this list.
- Fat provides more energy per gram (9 calories) than carbs (4 calories). Less equals more. You have to eat more than 2x the carbs to get the same energy as fat.
- Processed foods have more calories yet fewer nutrients. You get more fuel that you have to burn but fewer resources (nutrients) to give your body to work with.
- One of the biggest issues facing our society is chronic inflammation. The biggest causes of chronic inflammation are
  - Processed food
  - Excess carbs
  - Industrial seed oils (vegetable oil)
- The other major health issue many people deal with is insulin resistance, and the negative effect carbs have on people with Type 1 and Type 2 diabetes increases every year.

- Saturated fat is not bad for you. You need it for almost every function of your body.

Following a ketogenic, whole food, and animal-based diet removes all the crap inhibiting your metabolic function.

- It allows the body to start burning body fat for fuel.
- It increases the amount of nutrition you get each day
- It helps your metabolism by improving the accessibility of nutrients
- It removes factors that can adversely affect insulin resistance and cause diabetes
- It significantly reduces inflammation.
- It improves gut health and digestive issues.

With that list of things, I often wonder why everyone isn't doing it already. The number of things that we deal with daily because of carbohydrates affecting our bodies is mind-boggling.

That's just the beginning. It gets better.

With a ketogenic diet, we lose fat, improve overall bodily function, and help our bodies heal over time. Here's how:

1. The most bioavailable foods are meats. Also, the most highly nutritious food too. Less eating and calories, more nutrients
2. More fat is a huge benefit of the diet. 60%-70% of the food you eat will be fats. You'll feel full, have more energy, and your body will start to feel fresh again with more fat in your life.
3. Digestion issues usually go away. Again, less food, less waste. Less need for extra stuff to digest the food equals fewer digestion issues.
4. Easier to regulate gains and losses. Smaller changes in how much you eat can have a greater effect on your progress towards your goal.
5. There is no need for a lot of supplements. Eating real food provides real nutrition.

6. Reduce meal prep and the amount of time you spend thinking about food.

A ketogenic diet generally takes away the seriously bad stuff and replaces it with seriously good stuff. Your body will function better with less inflammation, less stress, and more energy to fuel your active lifestyle.

There are four basic concepts behind following a whole food, animal-based Ketogenic Diet.

1. Eat animal meat, eggs, and animal by-products because they have everything the human body needs to thrive.
2. Eliminate industrial seed oils (vegetable oils). They are poison and have no place in a human diet.
3. Processed foods and Carbs create inflammation in the human body and are the root cause of most if not all chronic issues we face today.
4. The human body is built to use fat as its primary source of fuel, not carbs.

The more you focus on eating animals, the more nutritious your meals will be and the less stress you'll put on your body.

The practical application of this concept is reducing your carb intake, focusing on getting adequate protein and enough fat to fuel your body efficiently.

Removing processed food, seed oils, and carbs from your diet teaches your body how to use fat as its main fuel and reduces most of the things that are causing your body stress.

You are simultaneously improving your body's performance and removing things that hinder your performance. Double Win!!

Note: You'll notice I didn't say anything about testing ketones or being in Ketosis. Don't waste your time or money on any of that.

These four concepts are the basis for why a whole food, animal-based Ketogenic Diet works. I'll go over more about Ketosis and ketones in the "Common myths get busted" section of the book.

Step One

Commit to a time and stick with it.

Everyone is different. When I started, I did it overnight, 100%, and never looked back. I have worked with others who need to make the changes in small steps. Whichever way works best for you is fine. The more important factor is giving yourself a timeframe to make the changes and see how they affect you.

That's a hard one. Many people are not patient enough. Here's an expectation for you to have. It could take up to 6 months to see some changes based on your reason and what you're looking for. Many people report improved energy, fewer body aches, fat loss, and other changes..., anywhere from 3 weeks to 8 weeks. Major healing from hormone imbalances, autoimmune and other issues can take longer.

When I work with someone, it's for a minimum of 8 weeks. In my experience, it takes that long for most people to get the hang of the protocol and build a routine around it. I wouldn't suggest anyone change to an animal-based diet for less than eight weeks. Ideally, 90 days would give you a more realistic idea of how your body will function, especially if you're an active person who regularly exercises or plays a sport.

Step Two

Decide what to eat.

There are two parts to this step. The first part is deciding how far you want to go. Do you want to jump straight in, or do you want to take it one step at a time? The second part is deciding what to eat.

If you want to take it a step at a time, that's fine. Just remember your results are directly tied to how much you adhere to the diet.

Here are the guidelines for what to eat on a ketogenic, whole food, and animal-based diet.

1. Food that is as close to its natural form as possible. **If it has an ingredient label, it's not real food.**
2. Animal-based food. Preferable ruminants and red meat.
3. Dairy is optional. Some people can tolerate it. Most people do better without it.
4. Coffee and spices are usually ok. (as close to their natural form as possible)

There are plenty of options here. I've been following these guidelines for four years. Not once have I ever been bored or gotten tired of it.

Step Three

Figure out how much to eat.

Here comes the macro talk. Most people dread this part. Counting calories and measuring every bite is why many people quit following a Ketogenic Diet. I don't do calories, and I don't think you should measure your food for a living.

I do want you to weigh and measure for as long as it takes you to get comfortable with eyeballing your food and having a good idea of 1. how much it is, and 2. what it takes to make you feel satisfied at a meal. Once you have a handle on what proper amounts look and feel like, you should only need to measure again if you want to make a change and need to reset your "feelers".

I keep macros simple. Figure out your lean mass. Convert it to grams. Eat AT LEAST that much protein. Eat NO MORE than that much Carbs and Fat combined. That's it. You only need to worry about one number.

If you weigh 250lbs. and you're 30% body fat, you have about 175lbs. of lean mass. Your macros are 175 grams of protein *minimum* and 175 grams carbs/fat *or less* each day. If you're mixing your carbs and fat into the combined 175 grams, make sure you get at least 70g of fat each day. Your body needs it.

This graphic shows how it all works out.

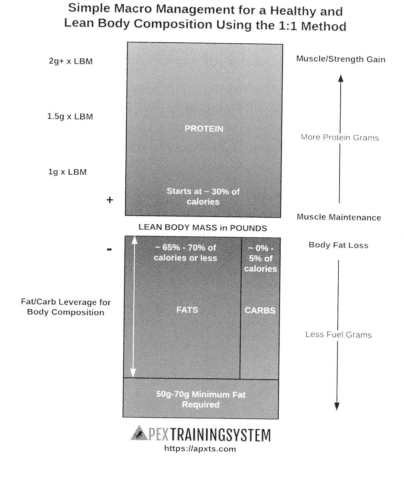

Figure 15 - 1:1 Macro Management

Step Four

Supplement properly.

You need to have a good clean diet for supplements to do what they're supposed to. Good thing you're going ketogenic!!

There are a handful of basic supplements that everyone should be taking regardless of the way of eating they follow. Call it a side-effect of the industrial age, but we don't get the micronutrients and minerals we need like we did when we lived off the earth and hunted our food.

It's important to get these because as you clean up your body, it will start working better, and it will need all the pieces of the puzzle to heal and improve.

The number one thing you need to do is start adding more salt to your food. Many people respond best with 3 grams - 5 grams per day. Some people need more. I do about 8 grams a day. Salt helps with energy and digestion.

I use either Drink LMNT (@drinklmnt) or Redmond Re-Lyte (@redmondrealsalt) for my electrolytes. They both have great flavor, and the combinations of minerals are just about perfect. I do 4-6 servings a day

Other recommended supplements:

- Vitamin D
- Zinc
- Magnesium
- Omega 3's (fish oil)

Step Five

Know what to expect.

Keto Flu When you first start reducing carbs in your diet, your body has to adapt. Carb withdrawal can cause "flu-like" symptoms and make some people tired, sore, and irritable. It usually lasts for a few days then goes away as your body adapts to using fat for fuel.

Bowel Movements You may have either loose or difficult bowel movements. Make sure to increase your sodium and electrolyte intake to help with this. It should get better in a week or two. You can expect to have fewer bowel movements with less volume. It doesn't mean you are constipated. There's just less to get rid of.

The best thing to do for each of these issues is to hydrate and increase your sodium and electrolyte intake.

Mindset and Belief System There will be changes in how your food affects your body, which may be challenging for you to understand. You should feel less hungry after each meal. You won't need to eat as many meals. You may realize that you've been starving yourself to reduce calories, and you need to eat more to get healthy. Removing carbs is not easy. They are addicting.

Go into this transition with a goal, and commit to a timeframe. Be open-minded about the process. Ask for help if you need it. The changes to your diet are pretty straightforward. The mental shift and learning how to build sustainable habits is where coaching and mentoring become a lifesaver.

Step Six

Decide what's next.

Assuming you've stuck with it for your intended timeframe, what's next? Do you keep going, or do you start to add more carbs back in to see what happens?

I just kept going. I'm very glad I did. My food prep is easy, my shopping is easy and cheap, and I rarely think about food throughout the day. I cannot deny the physical and mental improvements I've seen in my life. I don't see any reason why I would want to go back to feeling the way I used to.

Transitioning back to some carbs can be tricky. Why would you want to go back to the things that were causing you issues and reducing your ability to enjoy life?

- Defining your goal has to be number one at all times. Every choice you make needs to answer the question. "Will this help me reach my goal?"
- Don't decide to do something that adds to your stress and decreases your chance of sticking with the plan.
- Associate with people doing the same thing. Find groups where you can get support, information, recipes, and other social interaction from people who have similar goals.
- Get a coach. Nothing is more effective than working with a professional who has the experience and can help you work through your specific challenges.

Choose your carbs wisely

Avoiding carbs can be a challenge because there are so many options. The first thing to remember is that all carbs are plants. When we're talking about eating carbs, we're talking about choosing which plants we want to eat. Plants are a bit more complicated for humans than you may realize.

Let's take the whole carbohydrate thing off the table and just talk about plants.

When you are choosing what to eat besides the meat on your plate, there are a few things you need to evaluate.

1. Digestion
2. Inflammation
3. Anti-Nutrients
4. Bioavailability

Digestion

Plant digestion is a lot of work. The things needed to properly break down plants are pretty long. The main reason for this is a substance called Cellulose.

Cellulose is a complex carbohydrate. It makes up 33% of all plant matter on average (cotton is 90% cellulose, wood is 50%).

The human body has zero ability to break down cellulose. On average, 33% of the plants you eat provide no nutritional or energy benefit to your body.

Other animals have plenty of tools that make them much better plant-eaters. For example, cows have things that make them very efficient at turning plants into meat.

- Very long digestive system (small intestine and colon)

- Specific enzymes for digestion of plants (none for protein)
- Teeth designed for extreme mastication and physical breakdown of plants
- Regurgitation for extended mastication and digestion
- Fermentation of plant material before digestion

Humans don't have any of these. Our digestive system is smaller, and while it will support some ingestion of plants, it is not optimized.

The ability to breakdown plants at some level is a great example of the flexibility and adaptability of the human body. However, just because it can do something doesn't mean it's great at it.

Digesting plants is intensive and creates internal stress in the body.

Inflammation

Inflammation is the result of stress or injury. When you scratch your arm, it turns red and gets puffy. That's inflammation. When we eat a lot of things that make our body do extra work, it decreases the overall performance of our metabolism.

Here are a few ways that inflammation increases the more plants we eat.

- Increased oxidative stress and the production of free radicals
- Increased cortisol levels elevate blood sugar and reduce insulin sensitivity.
- Chronic hormone imbalances.

There is a preponderance of chronic illness today, and high levels of ongoing inflammation are largely to blame.

Anti-Nutrients

Anti-Nutrients are in a variety of plant foods. They interfere with the absorption of vitamins, minerals, and other nutrients. They even get in the way of digestive enzymes, which are key for proper absorption.

There are a lot of them. They affect people to various extents based on individual biology, overall intake, and length of exposure. For some of them, the effects can be reduced by how the food is prepared. Still, many people have a negative reaction to anti-nutrients regardless.

Table 2 - Anti-Nutrients

Name	Effect	Food
Phytate	Interferes with mineral absorption.	Grains and Legumes
Gluten	Hard to digest, plant protein. It's an enzyme inhibitor that causes gastrointestinal distress.	Grains, some processed foods, and beer
Tannins	Enzyme inhibitors can cause protein deficiency.	Plant-based proteins, legumes, grains, and some fruits
Oxalates	Interferes with mineral absorption. The main cause of kidney stones and gout.	Legumes, leafy greens, and some grains.
Lectins	Reduces nutrient absorption and binds to the walls of the digestive system. Possible cause of some autoimmune disorders.	Grains and legumes

Saponins	Mineral and enzyme inhibitor linked to leaky gut and autoimmune disorders	Legumes (Soy), some vegetables, and some grains
Trypsin Inhibitor	Inhibits protease and reduces protein digestion.	Grains and legumes (Soy)
Isoflavones	Phytoestrogen may have benefits in small doses but negatively affects estrogen and the endocrine system if over-consumed.	Legumes (Soy)
Solanine	Beneficial in many cases, unless over-consumed or eaten by someone sensitive to "nightshades".	Nightshades
Chaconine	Beneficial and has anti-fungal properties unless over-consumed. Can cause digestive issues.	Corn and potatoes

NOTE: The more processed a food is, the more negative impact the anti-nutrients have over any potential benefit the original, whole food may have provided. Processing reduces nutrition and increases the calories and inflammatory response of food.

There's a lot to "digest" here (pun intended). An important take-away from the anti-nutrient discussion is how they affect the main reason we eat in the first place, getting nutrients into our body.

Bioavailability

Bioavailability is one of the biggest misunderstood concepts in nutrition today.

The food you eat is only as beneficial as your body's ability to access and use whatever nutrition it provides.

Too often, people eat food that is low in nutritional value, to begin with. When you add in the inflammatory response to carbs and processed foods, increase the difficulty of digesting what you eat, and pile on the effect of anti-nutrients., is it any wonder people are overfed and undernourished?!

Much of what you are eating is not making it into your body.

The biggest change you can make on your journey to health and a better quality of life is to change your focus to getting the most benefit and nutritional value from everything you eat. The bioavailability of the food you eat matters very, very much.

Improve your options

I know this all sounds bad for plants and, in turn, carbs. Honestly, it is pretty bad. There isn't much need for them in a healthy diet. However, they provide flavor, color, and variety to our food palate. Many people like them and want to keep them in their lives for one reason or another.

Here are some things you can do to include carbs in your diet without too much trouble.

1. If it bothers you, stop eating it. You have to take the time to test different things out and see if they affect you.
2. Pre-breakdown (fermentation and cooking) all plant food. The less raw it is, the less active the anti-nutrients are.
3. If it has an ingredient label, it's not food. Don't eat it.
4. Eat more red meat. Some things you may not know about red meat;
    a. Meat is the most nutritious food by quantity
    b. Meat is the most digestible food
    c. Meat has the highest bioavailability

If you increase your red meat intake, you may have room for some less nutrient-dense options without as much risk of going under-nourished.

Choosing what carbs to include in your diet can be a challenge. The process is mostly trial and error. Understanding what you're dealing with is a big step in making the ketogenic diet work for you.

Vitamins and minerals on a ketogenic diet

How can you consider yourself eating a healthy diet if you're not getting the nutrients you need from fruits and vegetables?

The thought that all the essential vitamins and minerals a body needs are found in just meat is often a leap too far for people to make.

But it's true.

There are 14 Vitamins and 16 Minerals essential to the human body.

Table 3 - Vitamins and Minerals

RETINOIDS AND CAROTENE (vitamin A; includes retinol, retinal, retinyl esters, and retinoic acid and are also referred to as "preformed" vitamin A. Beta-carotene can easily be converted to vitamin A as needed.)	Essential for vision, Lycopene may lower prostate cancer risk. Keeps tissues and skin healthy. Plays an important role in bone growth and the immune system. Diets rich in the carotenoids alpha-carotene and lycopene seem to lower lung cancer risk. Carotenoids act as antioxidants. Foods rich in the carotenoids lutein and zeaxanthin may protect against cataracts	Many people get too much preformed vitamin A from food and supplements. Large amounts of supplemental vitamin A (but not beta-carotene) can be harmful to bones.

THIAMIN (vitamin B1)	Helps convert food into energy. Needed for healthy skin, hair, muscles, and brain and is critical for nerve function.	Most nutritious foods have some thiamin.
RIBOFLAVIN (vitamin B2)	Helps convert food into energy. Needed for healthy skin, hair, blood, and brain	Most Americans get enough of this nutrient.
NIACIN (vitamin B3, nicotinic acid)	Helps convert food into energy. Essential for healthy skin, blood cells, brain, and nervous system	Niacin occurs naturally in food and can also be made by your body from the amino acid tryptophan with the help of B6.
PANTOTHENIC ACID (vitamin B5)	Helps convert food into energy. Helps make lipids (fats), neurotransmitters, steroid hormones, and hemoglobin	Deficiency causes burning feet and other neurologic symptoms.
PYRIDOXINE (vitamin B6, pyridoxal, pyridoxine, pyridoxamine)	Aids in lowering homocysteine levels and may reduce the risk of heart disease helps convert tryptophan to niacin	Many people don't get enough of this nutrient.

and serotonin, a neurotransmitter that plays key roles in sleep, appetite, and moods. Helps make red blood cells Influences cognitive abilities and immune function

COBALAMIN (vitamin B12)

Aids in lowering homocysteine levels may lower the risk of heart disease. Assists in making new cells and breaking down some fatty acids and amino acids. Protects nerve cells and encourages their normal growth. Helps make red blood cells and DNA

Some people, particularly older adults, are deficient in vitamin B12 because they have trouble absorbing this vitamin from food. Those on a vegan or vegetarian diet often don't get enough B12as it's mostly found in animal products. They may need to take supplements. A lack of vitamin B12 can cause memory loss, dementia, and numbness in the arms and legs.

BIOTIN	Helps convert food into energy and synthesize glucose. Helps make and break down some fatty acids. Needed for healthy bones and hair	Bacteria make some in the gastrointestinal tract. However, it's not clear how much of this the body absorbs.
ASCORBIC ACID (vitamin C)	Foods rich in vitamin C may lower the risk for some cancers, including the mouth, esophagus, stomach, and breast. Long-term use of supplemental vitamin C may protect against cataracts. Helps make collagen, a connective tissue that knits together wounds and supports blood vessel walls. Helps make the neurotransmitters serotonin and norepinephrine Acts as an antioxidant, neutralizing unstable molecules that can damage cells. Bolsters the immune system	Evidence that vitamin C helps reduce colds has not been convincing.

CHOLINE	Helps make and release the neurotransmitter acetylcholine, which aids in many nerve and brain activities. Plays a role in metabolizing and transporting fats	Normally the body makes small amounts of choline. But experts don't know whether this amount is enough at certain ages.
CALCIFEROL (vitamin D)	Helps maintain normal blood levels of calcium and phosphorus, which strengthen bones. Helps form teeth and bones. Supplements can reduce the number of non-spinal fractures	Many people don't get enough of this nutrient. While the body uses sunlight to make vitamin D, it cannot make enough if you live in northern climates or don't spend much time in the sun.
ALPHA-TOCOPHEROL (vitamin E)	Acts as an antioxidant, neutralizing unstable molecule that can damage cells. Protects vitamin A and certain lipids from damage. Diets rich in vitamin E may help prevent Alzheimer's disease.	Vitamin E does not prevent wrinkles or slow other aging processes.

FOLIC ACID (vitamin B9, folate, folacin)

Vital for new cell creation helps prevent brain and spine birth defects when taken early in pregnancy; should be taken regularly by all women of child-bearing age since women may not know they are pregnant in the first weeks of pregnancy. It can lower homocysteine levels and may reduce heart disease risk. May reduce the risk for colon cancer. Offsets breast cancer risk among women who consume alcohol

Many people don't get enough of this nutrient. Occasionally, folic acid masks a B12 deficiency, leading to severe neurological complications. That's not a reason to avoid folic acid; just be sure to get enough B12.

PHYLLOQUINONE, MENADIONE (vitamin K)

Activates proteins and calcium essential to blood clotting. It may help prevent hip fractures

Intestinal bacteria make a form of vitamin K that accounts for half your require-ments. If you take an anti-coagulant, keep your vitamin K intake consistent.

CALCIUM	Builds and protects bones and teeth. Helps with muscle contractions and relaxation, blood clotting, and nerve impulse transmission. Plays a role in hormone secretion and enzyme activation. Helps maintain healthy blood pressure	Adults absorb roughly 30% of calcium ingested, but this can vary depending on the source. Diets very high in calcium may increase the risk of prostate cancer.
CHLORIDE	Balances fluids in the body. A component of stomach acid, essential to digestion	New recommendations (DRIs) for chloride are under development by the Institute of Medicine.
CHROMIUM	Enhances the activity of insulin, helps maintain normal blood glucose levels, and is needed to free energy from glucose	Unrefined foods such as brewer's yeast, nuts, and cheeses are the best sources of chromium, but brewer's yeast can sometimes cause bloating and nausea, so you may choose

		to get chromium from other food sources.
COPPER	Plays an important role in iron metabolism and the immune system. Helps make red blood cells	More than half of the copper in foods is absorbed.
FLUORIDE	Encourages strong bone formation. Keeps dental cavities from starting or worsening	Harmful to children in excessive amounts.
IODINE	Part of thyroid hormone that helps set body temperature and influences nerve and muscle function, reproduction, and growth. Prevents goiter and a congenital thyroid disorder	Some countries add iodine to salt, bread, or drinking water to prevent iodine deficiencies.
IRON	Helps hemoglobin in red blood cells and myoglobin in muscle cells ferry oxygen throughout the body. Needed for chemical	Many women of childbearing age don't get enough iron. Women who do not menstruate

	reactions in the body and for making amino acids, collagen, neuro-transmitters, and hormones	probably need the same amount of iron as men. Because iron is harder to absorb from plants, experts suggest vegetarians get twice the recommended amount (assuming the source is food).
MAGNESIUM	Needed for many chemical reactions in the body Works with calcium in muscle contraction, blood clotting, and blood pressure regulation. Helps build bones and teeth	The majority of magnesium in the body is found in bones. If your blood levels are low, your body may tap into these reserves to correct the problem.
MANGANESE	Helps form bones. Helps metabolize amino acids, cholesterol, and carbohydrates	If you take supplements or have manganese in your drinking water, avoid exceeding the upper limit. Those with liver

		damage or whose diets supply abundant manganese should be especially vigilant.
MOLYBDENUM	Part of several enzymes, one of which helps ward off a form of severe neurological damage in infants that can lead to early death	Molybdenum deficiencies are rare.
PHOSPHORUS	Helps build and protect bones and teeth. Part of DNA and RNA. Helps convert food into energy. Part of phospholipids, which carry lipids in blood and help shuttle nutrients into and out of cells	Certain drugs bind with phosphorus, making it unavailable and causing bone loss, weakness, and pain.
POTASSIUM	Balances fluids in the body. Helps maintain a steady heartbeat and send nerve impulses. Needed for muscle contractions. A diet	Food sources do not cause toxicity, but high-dose supplements might.

	rich in potassium seems to lower blood pressure. Getting enough potassium from your diet may benefit bones	
SELENIUM	Acts as an anti-oxidant, neutralizing unstable molecule that can damage cells. Helps regulate thyroid hormone activity	Researchers are investigating whether selenium may help reduce the risk of developing cancer, but with mixed results.
SODIUM	Balances fluids in the body. Helps send nerve impulses. It is needed for muscle contractions. Impacts blood pressure. A precursor to Hydrochloric Acid and aids in digestion	Recommended 3g-5g per day
SULFUR	Helps form bridges that shape and stabilize some protein structures. Needed for healthy hair, skin, and nails	Sulfur is a component of thiamin and certain amino acids. There is no recommended

		amount for sulfur. Deficiencies occur only with a severe lack of protein.
ZINC	Helps form many enzymes and proteins and create new cells. Frees vitamin A from storage in the liver. Needed for immune system, taste, smell, and wound healing. When taken with certain antioxidants, zinc may delay the progression of age-related macular degeneration	Because vegetarians absorb less zinc, experts suggest that they get twice the recommended zinc requirement from plant foods.

What's missing?

There are thirty vitamins and minerals in all. You can find all but five in meat, fish, and eggs.

Seriously! Out of the five nutrients, we don't get from animal products, two we don't need anyway. One needs supplementation regardless of what diet you choose, and the other two we could use less of in most cases.

Table 4 - Micronutrients we do and don't need

ASCORBIC ACID (vitamin C)	Not needed in nearly as much quantity as we've been told so long as little to no carbohydrates are consumed.
CALCIFEROL (vitamin D)	Supplementation is usually required regardless of diet choice.
CHLORIDE	Supplementation with salt is needed on a whole food, animal-based Ketogenic Diet. Recommended 3-5mg per day
FLUORIDE	There is plenty of current debate about whether we need as much as we are now.
SODIUM	Supplementation with salt is needed on a whole food, animal-based Ketogenic Diet. Recommended 3-5mg per day

Meats and animal products have each vitamin and mineral at various levels. It's important to realize is that the recommendations (RDA or Recommended Daily Allowance) for each of these vitamins and minerals are derived from the Standard American Diet. The recommended amounts are based on a high-carb diet, with plant-based foods providing a large percentage of the nutrients.

Refer to the earlier information in the "Chose your carbs wisely" chapter and consider these recommendations in the light of that discussion. How bioavailable and nutrient-dense is the Standard American Diet?

Here's a great visual of the benefits of meat vs. plants. Meat is more bio-available and much more nutrient-dense than most plants.

NUTRIENTS IN "SUPERFOODS" COMPARED TO ANIMAL PROTEIN

Per Serving	Apples	Blueberries	Kale	Beef	Beef Liver
Calcium (mg)	9.1	4.5	63.4	9.7	9.7
Magnesium (mg)	7.3	4.5	15.0	16.7	15.8
Phosphorus (mg)	20.0	9.0	24.6	154.0	340.6
Potassium (mg)	163.8	57.8	200.6	325.6	334.4
Iron (mg)	0.2	0.2	0.8	2.9	7.7
Zinc (mg)	0.2	0.2	0.2	4.0	3.5
Selenium (mcg)	0.0	0.1	0.4	12.5	34.9
Vitamin A (IU)	69.2	40.5	13530.9	35.2	46992.0
Vitamin B6 (mg)	0.0	0.1	0.1	0.4	1.0
Vitamin B12 (mcg)	0.0	0.0	0.0	1.8	97.7
Vitamin C (mg)	7.3	7.3	36.1	1.8	23.8
Vitamin D (IU)	0.0	0.0	0.0	6.2	16.7
Vitamin E (mg)	0.2	0.5	0.8	1.5	0.6
Niacin (mg)	0.2	0.3	0.4	4.2	15.0
Folate (mcg)	0.0	4.5	11.4	5.3	127.6

Figure 16 - Plant Superfood vs. Animal Protein

If you are going Ketogenic and want to play it safe, include organ meats or supplements made from them. Beef liver, in particular, has the highest levels, per ounce, of most of the 30 essential vitamins and minerals. If you aren't a fan of cooking and eating liver, you can get powdered beef liver pills at most vitamin or supplement shops.

Summary

I have not seen any information that leads me to believe removing vegetables will cause any reduction in micronutrients that would pose a health risk, short or long term.

On the contrary, I have talked to and can refer to hundreds if not thousands of people that do not eat vegetables and have no health issues to show for it. You don't have to completely cut them out if you don't want to.

I just want you to know that there isn't a requirement for plants, and you need to understand the impact and how to mitigate any risk you may incur from eating them.

Old knowledge is hard to break, and new information takes time to verify and make popular. You make up your mind.

More about protein

Protein is a subject of much debate regarding its effect on the body, calories, and improving performance. The most common topics concerning protein fall under;

- Too much protein will kick you out of ketosis
- Too much protein will turn to fat

We need protein

After water, protein is the main component of cells and is essential to life. Your body uses protein to build and maintain many parts and functions in your body:

- Muscles are responsible for movement. Many organs are made of muscle, including your heart.
- Collagen Provides strength and structure to tissues (e.g., the cartilage in joints).
- Skin, hair, and nails are mainly composed of protein.
- Hemoglobin transports oxygen around the body.
- Hormones act as your body's chemical messengers.
- Enzymes regulate metabolism. They support important chemical reactions that allow you to digest food, generate energy to contract muscles, and regulate insulin production.
- Antibodies play a role in your immunity.

Being metabolically unhealthy changes the interaction

Protein is low on the glycemic index, which means it doesn't raise sugar on its own. It does, however, have a moderate effect on insulin. It raises insulin, similar in some cases, to carbs.

When someone is insulin resistant, has pre-diabetes, or type 2 diabetes, they could have a problem where anytime they eat ANYTHING, their blood sugar will go up.

Many people believe that eating too much protein will make them fat if they are insulin resistant because protein increases insulin and raises their blood sugar at the same time. The important thing to remember is that the problem is not protein. Protein is not kicking you out of ketosis. The problem is a damaged liver that's not functioning properly.

Even with the liver creating extra blood sugar, protein, by its slower digestion rate, reduces the impact of the increased insulin and alleviates much of this problem.

Note: In the big picture of making dietary changes, an overall reduction of carbohydrates will vastly improve insulin resistance more than almost any amount of protein will have a negative effect. Do not fear protein.

- Protein positively affects improved performance, body fat loss, and lean mass gain.
- Protein is the building block of everything you need for health and longevity.
- The insulinemic effect of protein assists with building and maintaining muscle.
- Protein is more satiating. You will feel full with fewer calories and stay full longer
- The more protein you eat, the hotter your body runs which could increase body fat loss (Thermogenesis)

How much should you eat?

What I recommend is 1 gram of protein per pound of lean mass or goal weight) for fat loss.

Over many years and many successful clients, I've never had an issue with someone having too much protein.

I will often recommend 1.5 grams per pound of lean mass for someone interested in improving performance.

Everything you do should start with a base of how much protein you need each day. Figure this out, then stick with it.

It's nearly impossible to eat too much protein

Paradigm shifts take time. Protein is not a fuel source. In the presence of carbs or fats, it's generally not used to create ATP for muscular activation.

When we look at oxidative priority, we find that protein is not a source of energy the body can easily use.

Energy Generated is not the same as Energy Utilized (Burned is not the same as Used)

Here's an analogy for you.

Your car utilizes/burns gasoline to make it move and get you from point A to point B. Your car generates energy in the form of heat that you need oil to help manage so it doesn't burn out. Oil is not a fuel, but it is essential to keep your car functioning efficiently.

When we talk about macronutrients, Carbs and Fats are the gasoline your body uses for fuel. Protein is the oil.

Protein can be burned for fuel if needed, but its main purpose is to help your body function properly (cellular repair and metabolic function). Your body heats up when you eat protein. That doesn't mean it's fuel.

What you didn't know about Oxidative Priority (Processing vs. Fueling)

Fuel Source	Alcohol	Exogenous Ketones	Protein	Carbohydrates	Fat	Protein
Oxidative Priority	1	2	3	4	5	6
Utilization	Energy	Energy	Cellular Repair and Metabolic Function	Energy	Energy	Energy/Excretion
Storage Capacity	Zero	Limited, a few grams	~120 grams	500 grams	Unlimited	Unlimited
Thermic Effect Cost	15%	Assumed to be 3%	35%	8%	3%	35%

1. Oxidative Priority is NOT linear, it's fluid
2. Rate of Storage vs. Utilization varies based on
   a. Metabolic health
   b. Activity level and volume
   c. Availability of fuel in total
   d. Availability of fuel by type
   e. Speed of digestion
3. The more adipose tissue you have, the more likely your body will try to store fat (white vs brown fat)
4. It takes around 1.6g of protein per pound of Lean Mass to create a break-even balance of protein the body COULD use for fuel if it was needed (Not accounting for activity level or other fuel sources available)
5. Several studies have shown minimal to zero body fat gain due to overfeeding of protein (up to 3g of protein per pound of lean mass)
6. These same studies have shown marked increase in Lean Mass in protein overfed individuals

It is almost impossible, at least, improbable that anyone would or could regularly eat enough protein to gain fat from it. Our bodies use protein to repair and build as the priority. As long as there is a need for cellular repair and metabolic function, protein will, likely, not be used for fuel.

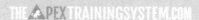

THE APEXTRAININGSYSTEM.COM

Figure 17 - Updated Oxidative Priority (Protein is different)

Targeting a % of calories for carbs, fat, and protein will set you up for a stall in fat loss and overall progress in many cases. I've seen it happen over and over again.

Total caloric intake is inaccurate because 1/3 of the total calories don't get used as fuel.

What if you just focused on the protein? What if we only counted from fats and carbs as fuel?!?!

Fuel Calories vs. Functional Calories

Eat protein to maintain metabolic function (functional calories). Leverage carbs and fat (fuel calories) to manage body composition.

This does a few things:

- It's usually more food than they're used to
- Increases satiety, so you get full faster and stay full longer
- There's less focus on adding fat to everything
- Being full means having fewer cravings
- Overall, fuel calories go down. (Whether total calories do or not)
- Improves body fat reduction
- Facilitates muscle preservation and growth
- Reduces stress around food and food choices

Protein builds muscles. Muscles burn fat. If you have excess body fat, let your body use it for fuel. If you are trying to lose fat, then stop eating more fat. It's that simple.

Common Myths Get Busted

There is a lot of information on fitness and nutrition available on the Internet. Thousands of people have been sharing research and personal experience for years and years. While this is amazing, and access to information is helpful to many, it also creates a bit of a problem.

The information is not always accurate. The context or applicability of the information is often misunderstood.

I've encountered several questions and beliefs that I think need to be addressed. The information in this section may be opposite what you think. That's good.

I want to challenge you to learn more and see if what I'm saying makes sense. What if these things are true? How does it change your approach or how you work to improve your quality of life?

Ketogenesis feeds Gluconeogenesis

If you're like many people in the keto community, you've heard plenty about gluconeogenesis (GNG). The most common discussion topics are about how too much protein can be detrimental to ketosis because gluconeogenesis will turn it into glucose and stop you from burning fat.

In general, the thought is that GNG is in competition with ketogenesis (KG) for energy production. Fat vs. Protein, in a never-ending battle.

What if it wasn't that way at all? What if GNG was, in fact, complementary to KG and enhanced the metabolic efficiency of being in a fat-burner?

Gluconeogenesis – The Basics

The dictionary definition of GNG is "formation of glucose within the animal body, especially by the liver from substances (such as fats and proteins) other than carbohydrate".

Notice "such as fats and proteins"?

Wait!!!! GNG can use fats to create glucose?!?!?!?!

Yes. GNG is not a specific, protein-driven process. It can use other substances to generate energy.

One of the biggest concerns with GNG is that protein consumption will increase glucose production. This isn't true. GNG doesn't rely on protein, and if there are other substances it can use, it will use them first. Protein metabolism is energy expensive. Protein is prioritized for muscle protein synthesis, cellular repair, metabolic function, and many other non-energy-related systems in the body. Your body doesn't want to use protein for fuel unless it needs to.

GNG is an umbrella term for all processes used to produce glucose for energy. Yes, there is more than one.

Gluconeogenesis – A little deeper

GNG uses four main substances. Three of them are byproducts of KG. One is amino acids.

- Acetate
- Pyruvate
- Lactate
- Glucogenic Amino Acids

There are two main cycles of metabolism GNG uses to create glucose from these four substances.

Krebs Cycle – Energy production with Oxygen

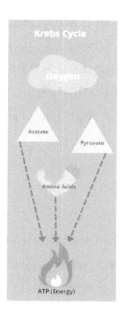

- Acetate
- Pyruvate
- Glucogenic Amino Acids

Pyruvic acid supplies energy to living cells through the Krebs cycle when oxygen is present (aerobic respiration); when oxygen is lacking, it ferments to produce lactic acid (lactate).

Cori Cycle – Energy production without Oxygen

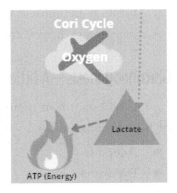

- Lactate

Anaerobic work creates lactate as a byproduct of glycolysis (the breakdown of muscle glycogen). Lactate is re-used in the Cori Cycle to create glucose.

Lactate is also a byproduct of the breakdown of Acetone from KG

Where do the other substances besides amino acids come from?

Acetate, Pyruvate, and Lactate come from ketogenesis.

What is Ketogenesis?

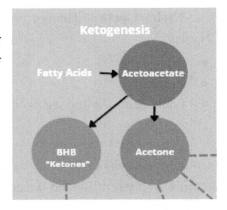

The dictionary definition of ketogenesis is "the production of ketone bodies."

Well, that's fairly anti-climatic.

The three ketone bodies created by KG are:

- Acetoacetate is the first ketone body and breaks up into the other two.
- B-hydroxybutyrate (BHB) is the most abundant ketone body, and it is the main source of fuel for the body. (commonly referred to as ketones)

- Acetone is not an "active" metabolite. It breaks down into Acetate, Pyruvate, and Lactate.

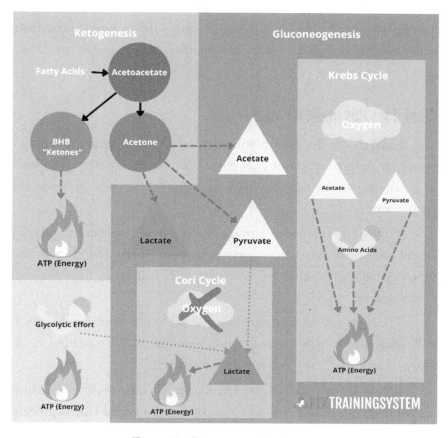

Figure 18 - Ketogenesis feeds Gluconeogenesis

The major benefits we get from KG are the abundance of BHB for fuel. Reducing carbohydrates as the main fuel source allows for BHB to take over. By producing and breaking down Acetone, keto-genesis facilitates the creation of the three metabolites added back into other energy cycles to create glucose.

Ketogenesis and Gluconeogenesis work together to provide either source of energy the body needs when it is needed. Being fat-adapted feeds BOTH ketone AND glucose production. GNG is happening all the time. Carbs are more of a risk of being in ketosis than protein

It's not one or the other. GNG doesn't necessarily cancel out ketosis. If you're fat-adapted and making sure to keep carbs from becoming the dominant source of fuel, then staying in ketosis should never be a problem.

What does this mean for you?

First, this is the reason you don't need to worry about eating a bunch of carbs to workout effectively. Your body is perfectly capable of producing all the fuel you need from the fat on your body and the fat you eat.

Your body's glycogen storage is more than sufficient to provide all the fuel you need for any workout you do. KG and GNG working together will easily replenish your glycogen storage in time for your next workout.

There's a reason carbs are considered non-essential nutrients. It is illogical to say that carbs are non-essential but are needed to do physical activity…. It's not factually consistent.

Secondly, you need to give the adaptation time to develop. There are three levels of adaptation you need to go through. Unfortunately, few people talk about this in the context of exercise and fitness.

Fat-adaptation is the process of teaching your body how to use fat more efficiently. The reduction or elimination of carbs forces your body to learn a new way of doing things. This takes 1-2 weeks. You may experience carb withdrawal (keto flu) and you won't have a ton of energy to do much if any activity, especially exercise.

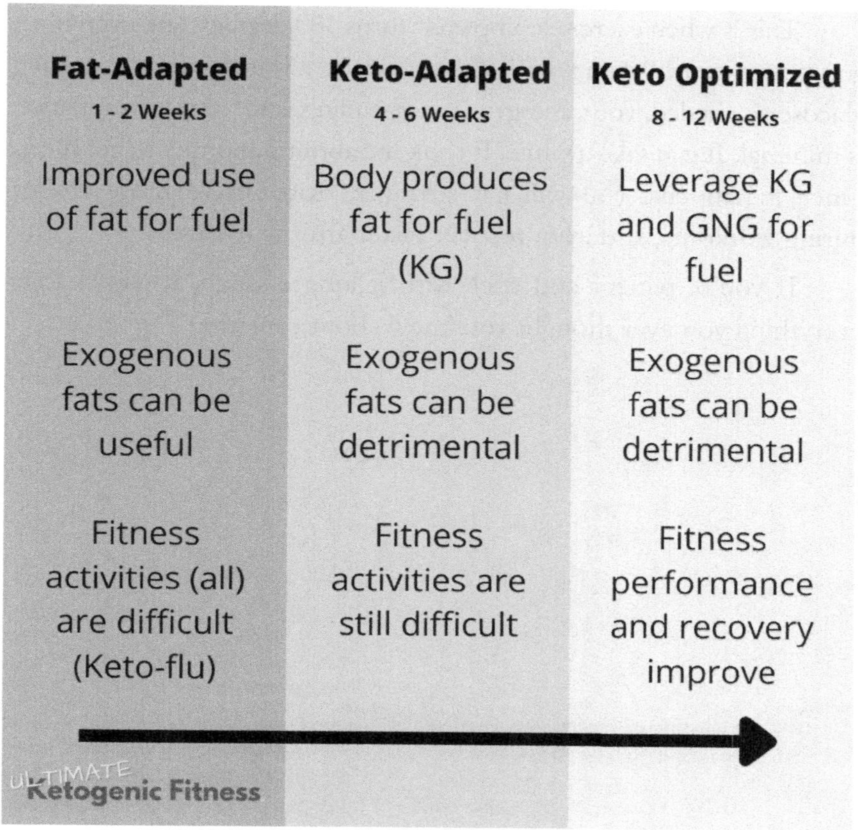

Fat-Adapted	Keto-Adapted	Keto Optimized
1 - 2 Weeks	4 - 6 Weeks	8 - 12 Weeks
Improved use of fat for fuel	Body produces fat for fuel (KG)	Leverage KG and GNG for fuel
Exogenous fats can be useful	Exogenous fats can be detrimental	Exogenous fats can be detrimental
Fitness activities (all) are difficult (Keto-flu)	Fitness activities are still difficult	Fitness performance and recovery improve

Ketogenic Fitness

Figure 19 - The progressions of Ketogenic adaptation

Keto-adaptation is the stage where your body is good at burning fat but is learning to produce its own fat fuels (ketones) without you needing to eat as much. This is often a stall point because your body is ready to use more of what is stored in body fat, but people tend to keep eating fat and blocking that transition. This process happens around the 4–6 week point. Normal day-to-day energy is usually good by this time, but exercise activities are still a challenge.

Keto-optimized is what I call the final stage of adaptation. It's where your body is efficient at not just fat utilization but also glucose creation. The interaction between Ketogenesis and Gluconeogenesis is the main fuel production process in use.

This is when exercise completely turns 180 degrees, and everything gets blown away! When your body is efficient at burning fat and making glucose as needed, your energy is never-ending, and your inflammation is minimal. It can take a while. It took me about 3 months to get there. Once it happens, you will get stronger, faster, have more energy during workouts, and even recover faster after workouts.

If you're patient and stick with it long enough, it will change everything you ever thought you knew about exercise.

Stop chasing Ketosis

Ketosis is often used as a defining characteristic of being in a state of Ketogenesis. Measuring your blood or urine ketone levels is a common method to tell you if you're burning fat for fuel.

Let's dig into that a little bit.

Ketosis is defined as a metabolic state where ketone levels are elevated in the blood or urine.

Ketogenesis is the production of ketones. The idea that if you are producing ketones, then you are going to have more ketones in your blood makes sense.

Here's the tricky part. Ketones are produced by the breakdown of fatty acids. No ketone testing exists that can tell you if the ketones showing up on your test strips came from body fat being metabolized or from the MCT oil and butter you just drank in your coffee.

It is possible and very common to be in a technical state of ketosis without utilizing body fat at all. That kind of defeats the point of following a Ketogenic Diet, doesn't it?

The first reason ketone testing and focusing on Ketosis can throw off your progress is because it's not a true indicator of where your fat fuel is coming from.

But wait, there's more!

Ketones are the main fuel used by the body when glycogen from carbs are reduced or eliminated.

If your body is using mostly ketones for fuel, why do you want high levels of them in your blood?

When we are carb fueled, high blood glucose is bad, causes inflammation and increases fat storage. It's excess fuel the body can't use.

How is excess fuel now beneficial just because it's fat? High ketones in your blood mean you have fuel that is not being used. What happens to fuel that is not used? It gets stored as body fat and increases inflammation.

This is another reason focusing on high ketones and being in Ketosis will keep you from reaching your goals. Your body may react and metabolize carbs and fats differently, but fuel is fuel. It's either used or stored. There's no way around that.

The benefits of following a whole food, animal-based Ketogenic Diet come from the removal of substances that cause inflammation, increase body fat, and decrease lean mass.

Think of it this way. If you've reduced or eliminated carbs, then your body has no choice but to burn fat. Why do you need to measure anything?

If you only put 93 octane fuel in your car, do you then need to test the exhaust to make sure your car is only using 93 octane fuel? What's the point?

If you focus on getting adequate protein, limiting carbs, and eliminating processed foods and seed oils you will be immensely more successful following this lifestyle.

Forget Ketosis. Focus on real food.

The cholesterol myth

The overwhelming confusion and variation of information regarding fat in our diets and its effect on cholesterol and mortality are even bigger than the debate over whether carbs are essential for health.

There is a lot of current science on this subject. There is an even larger body of clinical evidence and how diverging from the mainstream recommendations and widely held theories has helped millions of people improve their health and live longer.

Eating saturated fat can and often does increase your LDL. It doesn't lead to heart disease. LDL isn't "bad" fat like many people believe. In fact, on a Ketogenic Diet, LDL helps transport all those fat molecules around in your blood to get used up by your body when it needs fuel. It is not uncommon for a person on a healthy, Ketogenic Diet to have their LDL number go up as their body gets better at burning fat for fuel.

The real source of heart disease is inflammation and increased triglycerides in the body. High triglycerides are more directly linked to heart disease than LDL. Many studies show a positive correlation between carb intake, high triglycerides, and increased cardiovascular disease and mortality.

On a ketogenic, whole food, and animal-based diet, HDL and LDL tend to rise while reducing carbs lowers Triglycerides. If you're getting bloodwork, this is the trend you are looking for. Here are two things to look for that could signal that something is off. These are good markers for healthy cholesterol, fat metabolism, and lower inflammation level. Remember, you want movement in the right direction. It's not going to happen overnight.

- **Total Cholesterol to HDL-Cholesterol Ratio:** This is how abundant your LDL particles are. The lower your TC to your HDL, the better.

- **Triglyceride to HDL Cholesterol Ratio:** This is how many large LDL particles you have vs. small LDL particles. Higher levels of small LDL particles often indicate higher levels of inflammation. The lower your Triglycerides are to your HDL, the more large LDL particles you have and the better off you are.

Note: Not just the ratios are important. A growing body of evidence shows that low LDL could indicate an increased risk for heart disease. Yes, the very goal of current medical treatment could be doing the opposite of what it says it will do.

Further investigation into why the rates of cardiovascular disease, hypertension, diabetes, and other inflammatory and related metabolic syndromes ailments have increased significantly in the last 100 years points squarely at the dramatic increase in industrial seed oils. Since the advent of Crisco and other brands of seed oils, often called vegetable oils, there has been a positive relationship between rates of illness and consumption.

Take the data from an analysis of dietary trends in the United States since 1800:

Table 5 - Seed Oil Consumption Tied to Sickness

Food	Consumption/Availability Change
Processed Food (high concentration of seed oils)	Increased from <5% to >60%
Red Meat	Decreased from 44% to 21%
Industrial Seed Oils (margarine, shortening, cooking oils)	Increased by 91% - 329%
Butter and Lard	Decreased by 68%-78%

"In every year since 1900 except 1918, CVD accounted for more deaths than any other major cause of death in the United States" *(Rosamond et al., Heart disease, and stroke statistics-2008 update 2007)*

Since 1900 the deaths from heart disease have gone from 25,000 a year to over 700,000 a year. While animal fat (saturated fat) consumption has remained fairly consistent and" heart-healthy", industrial seed oil consumption has increased.

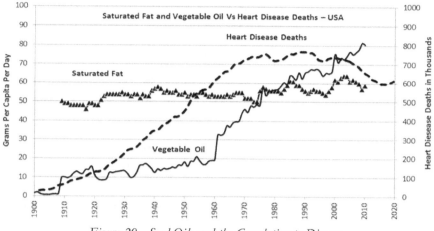

Figure 20 - Seed Oils and the Correlation to Disease

That's just the basics. Suffice it to say, everything you thought you knew about saturated fat and cholesterol is probably worth some further investigation. *(Hint; start in the references for this chapter)*

There have been books written about these topics. I'm not going to try and get that in-depth. There is scientific data out there and millions of people who are currently getting better and living longer by doing things differently.

I can't tell you what to do. Check all the references at the back of this book for more information. Do some research read some books. All I can say is that four years ago (May 2018), at 46 years old, I stopped eating seed oils and went to all fat from animals. My health, bloodwork, and life have only gotten better.

Salt is not the problem

"Don't put so much salt on your food!!"

I used to hear this all the time when I was a kid. I loved salt, but I was told it would kill me if I had too much.

Hypertension is a huge problem in the world today. Nearly half of the US population has high blood pressure!

What if I told you that salt doesn't cause hypertension?

In 2011, a study titled *"Urinary sodium and potassium excretion and risk of cardiovascular events"* evaluated almost 30,000 people over five years. Guess what they found?

The people that stayed closest to the current dietary guideline for sodium intake (2.3g or less per day) had the highest incidence of cardiovascular events. In contrast, those who had almost twice the recommended intake had fewer cardiovascular events!!!

What if I told that high blood pressure was caused by:

- Overconsumption of carbs and sugar
  - Sugar and carbs increase inflammation and dysregulate insulin in your body.
  - The more insulin resistant you become, the more hypertensive you become.
- Not getting enough Potassium
  - Potassium is important for muscle function and supports the electrical signals our central nervous system uses to communicate with all parts of the body.
  - Modern humans get about 2.5 grams of potassium per day. Before the industrial age, it's estimated that humans consumed upwards of 11 grams per day.
  - You are probably not getting enough potassium, especially if you aren't eating a fair amount of red meat.

- Not getting enough Magnesium
  - Magnesium is essential in regulating hundreds of metabolic processes like managing blood pressure, blood sugar regulations, energy production, and bone development.
  - Low Magnesium can also cause a "pseudo Potassium deficit" effect on your body.
  - Increasing Magnesium intake by as little as .5g a day has been shown to reduce hypertension.

Hypertension results from eating food that is low in micronutrients (low nutrient density) and high in carbs and processing (low bioavailability). It is a symptom of everything I've discussed that you need to avoid.

If these are the real reasons for hypertension, what is salt good for, and how much is too much?

Salt, particularly Sodium, is vital to the functioning of your body. It plays a role in cellular hydration. Sodium is a key component in extracellular fluid, blood, and lymph fluid.

Sodium is an integral part of the nervous system as it provides the mechanism by which neurons communicate with each other.

Sodium is the precursor to Hydrochloric Acid (HCL), the main acid responsible for breaking down food in your digestive tract.

As you can see, sodium plays a significant role in some vital components of how your body functions. Not having enough can be very detrimental to your health. You probably need more than you're getting right now.

I already mentioned the 2011 study that showed a higher risk of cardiovascular events with lower sodium intake. Common symptoms of inadequate sodium consumption are:

- Hypertension
- High triglycerides
- Insulin resistance/Diabetes
- Lethargy

- Increased bone injury
- Reduced cognitive function

Sodium is kind of a big deal. You probably need to start eating more. Leading health experts recommend 3 grams to 5 grams of sodium per day. I would lean more towards 5 grams, especially if you eat a ketogenic, whole food, and animal-based diet. The less sodium naturally in your food, the more you'll need to supplement.

I consume 9 grams to 11 grams of sodium per day if you need a reference. My blood pressure is good. I have more energy and feel generally better above 9 grams. I get my sodium primarily with 11 grams of Redmond's Real Salt (@redmonsrealsalt) on my food each day and 4-6 Drink LMNT or Redmond Re-Lyte electrolyte packets as part of my daily routine.

I know you've been told salt is bad. I hope the information I've laid out here is helping you to rethink and take a look at one more thing we've been misinformed about for a long time.

Cardio sucks for fat loss

I would rather you did 10 minutes of high intensity, full-body movement with weight than jog or ride a bike or elliptical for an hour.

Excessive cardio to lose body fat is a remnant of an old way of thinking. I am doing everything I can to help you let go of it.

Fat loss is not the goal. Fixing your metabolism is the goal.

Cardio is a tool used in a well-rounded program to help improve one of the metabolic pathways. But only one of them. There are still two more. There are also seven essential movements and ten components of fitness.

Cardio only addresses 3 of the 20 aspects of health and fitness you could be working on.

When you work out, you are improving the ability of your body to do something. When you lift weights, you get stronger, and they become easier to move. When you do cardio, the same thing happens. You get faster. You can go longer. You get better at conserving and using fuel. Cardio becomes easier.

This process means that the more cardio you do, the less fat you burn when you do it. Focusing on cardio at the expense of functional fitness has a steep rate of diminishing returns.

Cardio exercises only work while you are doing them. If I was trying to lose fat, cardio would not be my preferred method. I would do activities that used my whole body, add resistance, and increased the intensity of how hard I worked.

Functional movement at high intensity provides a more significant benefit to your fitness than cardio alone. Building lean mass is a great way to keep the fat burn going even when you aren't working out.

If you're stuck in the cardio trap and it makes up most of your exercise, it's time to step out of your comfort zone. If you don't challenge your body in different ways, you will be stuck in the same place year after year.

Ask youself, "How is this cardio helping me improve my _____?" You can use any of the following to fill in the blank.

- Strength
- Stamina
- Flexibility
- Agility
- Coordination
- Balance
- Speed
- Power
- Accuracy
- Squatting
- Hinging
- Lunging
- Pushing
- Pulling
- Twisting

I'm not saying you shouldn't do cardio; it's necessary. You shouldn't do it to the exclusion of other components of fitness. Go back to the Chapter "What to look for in a fitness program" and find out what you should be doing instead.

It's ok to get off the treadmill and go grab a weight. You can thank me later.

Bio-hacks probably aren't worth it

I'm using this last chapter as a catch-all for a handful of topics commonly discussed and debated in the Keto/Carnivore community. This book is not the place to expound on the scientific theories or mechanisms of how these unique tactics function or how to apply them, but I do want to address them.

I'm talking about bio-hacks. I don't think most people reading this book need to use them.

If you are metabolically unhealthy, you have enough on your plate. You're already working to establish good habits, listen to your body, eat enough protein, start exercising, meal prep, and make lifestyle changes.

You need to focus on the basics. Just focus on the basics.

Focus on the basics until you can do them with your eyes closed.

I will recommend that you get really good at these before you start bio-hacking

- Nutrient Density
- Bioavailability
- Satiety
- Functional Movement
- Intensity
- Recovery and Sleep

Becoming a pro at these six things will do far more for you than the stress and overhead of learning to do them and throwing in:

- One Meal A Day (OMAD)
- Extended Fasting

- Protein Sparing Modified Fast (PSMF)
- Carb cycling
- Nutrient timing
- Fasted workouts

In the years I have been coaching, I have not had a single person who used a bio-hack see success from the hack that they wouldn't have seen if they had locked in the basics first. Many people lost time, got stressed out, and even gave up because things were overwhelming. If they had kept it simple and focused on the basics, it would have been a much better experience.

When you get impatient, you want to try something that will speed up the process. Nothing works faster than sticking with the basics. Bio-hacks can have their place, but it's not usually while you're still healing and learning to live a whole new way of life.

Real People, Real Results

Here is a sample of what is happening to people following the guidance in this book. Some of these are clients who I have worked with one-on-one. Others were part of group challenges or subscribers to my online fitness program. Some of these people just listened to my content and tried some of the things I've talked about.

If it can work for these people, maybe, there's something here for you.

NOTE: If you want to get in on the fun, go to **https://ultimate-ketogenicfitness.com/sharing,** and you can add your story to the growing number of people whose lives are being changed by what's in this book!

"From about age 17 to 42, my health (and quality of life) slowly deteriorated. At 42, after having to go to the ER because I could not eat and I was vomiting blood, I was finally referred to a specialist to determine what was wrong. It was found, through an elimination diet, that I reacted to soy. However, I did not (and still do not) test positive for being allergic to soy. When I was 47, I was to a point where I could barely walk. I had to have knee surgery to repair an injury that occurred when I was 14 that went ignored by doctors. When I was 49, I woke up on Christmas Eve and could barely move my legs. I knew I had to do something.

On Christmas Eve, when I was 49, I decided that I needed to make a drastic change. I told my husband that I was going to start a

Ketogenic diet to cleanse my body and try to become healthy. By improving my nutrition through Keto, and now Keto-vore/Carnivore, I'm walking much better. I'm recovering from illnesses and injuries much faster. I went from barely being able to move my legs to walk 19K+ steps at a trade show in Las Vegas in 2 years. Not only that, but I recovered from that excessive walking faster than my husband did, and he's on his feet most of the day when he covers our store. My improved nutrition has made me healthier and stronger.

Fitness is a vital element in my life. When there is a lack of activity in my life, I become moody, depressed, and on edge. Not fun to be around. I used to be an avid gym-goer pre-Covid, but to be honest, I was mostly doing the same movements with the same equipment 3-4 days a week. I had no structure, no routine, and worst of all, no goals, but I enjoyed the feeling of working out. That is why Ultimate Ketogenic Fitness has been such a game-changer for me. It's such a great balance of strength training and high-intensity cardio, but more importantly for me, it's fun. I enjoy it. From the routines to the community, there is a sense we are part of something bigger, and that is motivating in itself. The endorphin rush received from completing a good workout is the highlight of my day. I am treating myself the best I ever have by pushing through mental and physical barriers." **– Theresa S.**

"As a 48-year-old CrossFitter, I am always looking for ways to improve strength and endurance. Enter the Carnivore diet. I have to say, I was skeptical at first, but I committed to it and am so happy I did. After a few short weeks, I saw myself get leaner, and my endurance improved. In the weeks to follow, I started hitting new PRs (Personal Records). I just noticed that I felt so much more energetic during my workouts. By 12 weeks, I had dropped 14 pounds and had PR'd almost every lift, and I felt great. It is an understatement to say I went from skeptic to advocate." **– Jason S.**

"I've been doing online training with Coach Dant since about May of 2020. I chose this program primarily because I am keto and wanted a Coach who understood and supported that way of eating - not one that would tell me I "needed" carbs to meet my goals.

I cannot suggest him more strongly. Need a modification? Aren't sure you are doing a movement correctly? All you have to do is reach out, send a video, whatever, and he responds right away. He's supportive of your goals and mindful of your needs when working with you.

In just under a year, I've lost 8lbs of fat and gained 7lbs of muscle. I've gone down two clothing sizes. I feel amazing, and I am getting stronger every day. I will also say the online workout community is an amazing group that will always cheer you on and asks what's going on if you are missing for a while - having a supportive community to keep you accountable, especially when you are working out solo - is invaluable!" **– Deanna H.**

"I'm so pumped to continue this journey with you guys. I know I was thinking of myself as an athlete in the past tense. This program is changing that. Now I know I can reach my health, fitness, body composition, and lifestyle goals while being a dad and running a business. More so than just my body changing, my outlook has changed. I'm looking forward to being a total badass, even when I'm as old as Bronson!" **– Matt S.**

"At one point, I was in super shape (26 years old, I'm 47 now) that date keeps getting farther and farther away. Every single year I set a goal to "get back in shape" before my birthday for that year! I had the idea to do it but never really made a plan or changed things. I just did more of what I was doing, run more, ride my bike more, swim more, or go to the gym more, and since I was "working out more," I could afford all the extra candy, beer, pizza calories right?! Wrong! I saw Bronson's post on Facebook, looking for seven guys to take on this challenge. I immediately emailed him because I saw the huge value in a COACH and a PLAN to get to a goal. I was afraid the class would be full already. I quickly asked my wife, if I made this commitment would she be able to continue to run our business effectively? Needless to say, she gave me her full support, and I signed up that day!... It's inspiring to see all of us getting better every day! Let's finish strong and then realize we didn't finish. We are just getting started!!!! Thanks for putting this all together, Bronson, and helping us realize our goals!" **– Neal S.**

"So I came into this program looking to lose weight... Joining this program has been awesome. My lungs are opening back up again, and I am using muscles that have been idle for a while. My day-to-day is very sedentary. So I am glad to be back in motion again. I am pleased to say that I have learned that the simplest diet change can affect your whole body. Not only have I lost weight, but I was able to reduce my blood pressure medicine from 320mg once a day to 40mg once a week. I am looking forward to the next four weeks with you guys." **– Boddrick H.**

"The quality of my life and health has changed SIGNIFICANTLY since I started the ketogenic diet in 2017. In the years prior, I was sick and overweight, and I felt hopeless. I had been overweight my entire life, and I was diagnosed with Crohn's Disease in 2015. When my Crohn's Disease was at its worst, I remember being in so much pain that I couldn't even stand up straight. Since starting Keto in 2017, I've been able to lose body fat and significantly reduce the inflammation in my body. Now that I'm no longer in pain, I can do anything! These days, I love dancing, traveling, lifting weights, and participating in the everyday joys of life!" – **Autumn W.**

"Fitness is a vital element in my life. When there is a lack of activity in my life, I become moody, depressed, and on edge. Not fun to be around. I used to be an avid gym-goer pre-Covid, but to be honest, I was mostly doing the same movements with the same equipment 3-4 days a week. I had no structure, no routine, and worst of all, no goals, but I enjoyed the feeling of working out. That is why Ultimate Ketogenic Fitness has been such a game-changer for me. It's such a great balance of strength training and high-intensity cardio, but more importantly for me, it's fun. I enjoy it. From the routines to the community, there is a sense we are part of something bigger, and that is motivating in itself. The endorphin rush received from completing a good workout is the highlight of my day. I am treating myself the best I ever have by pushing through mental and physical barriers." – **Glenn P.**

Continue Reading

This book is a collection of lessons learned, experiments I've done, and specific research I've conducted over the last ten years. I want you to start thinking outside the box, unlearn what you think you know, and be open to the possibility that your struggles with health are more about poor information than poor execution.

I hope that what you've read in this book has awakened your desire to learn more about health, nutrition, and fitness. Here are some of the best books you can read (or listen to) that will dig into every glorious detail and help you understand what's going on in your body.

Berry, K. D. (2019). Lies my doctor told me medical myths that can harm your health. Victory Belt Publishing Inc.

Emmerich, M., & Emmerich, C. (2018). Keto. The Complete Guide to success on the ketogenic diet, including simplified science and no-cook meal plans. Victory Belt Publishing Inc.

Naiman, T., & Shewfelt, W. (2020). The P:E diet: Leverage your biology to Achieve Optimal Health.

Rippetoe, M. (2007). *Strong enough?* The Aasgaard Company.

Cho, J. M., & Berry, K. D. (2020). Carnivore cure: The ultimate elimination diet to attain Optimal Health and heal your body. Nutrition with Judy.

BIKMAN, B. E. N. J. A. M. I. N. (2021). Why we get sick: The hidden epidemic at the root of most chronic disease and how to fight it. BENBELLA BOOKS.

Rippetoe, M., & Bradford, S. E. (2017). *Starting strength: Basic barbell training.* Aasgaard Company.

Taubes, G. (2007). *Good calories bad calories.* Gary A. Knopf.

Teicholz, N. (2014). *Big fat surprise.* Scribe Publications.

Cook, G. (2017). Movement: Functional movement systems: Screening, Assessment and Corrective Strategies. On Target Publications.

Fung, J. (2016). The obesity code: Unlocking the secrets of Weight Loss. Scribe.

Fung, J., & Teicholz, N. (2018). The diabetes code: Prevent and reverse type 2 diabetes naturally. Greystone Books.

Taubes, G. (2005). Big fat lie?: What if fat doesn't make you fat. Vermilion.

Simmons, L. (2015). Special strength development for all sports. Westside Barbell.

Saladino, P., & Sisson, M. (2020). The Carnivore Code: Unlocking the secrets to Optimal Health by returing to our ancestral diet. Fundamental Press.

Baker, S. (2020). *The carnivore diet.* Victory Belt Publishing.

Paoli, C., & Sherbondy, A. (2014). Free+style: Maximize sport and life performance with four basic movements. Victory Belt Publ.

PERLMUTTER, D. A. V. I. D. (2014). Grain brain: The surprising truth about wheat, carbs, and sugar - your brain's silent. Hodder & stoughton ltd.

Volek, J. S., & Phinney, S. D. (2012). *The art and science of low carbohydrate performance.* Beyond Obesity LLC.

Wolfe, L. (2013). Eat the yolks: Discover paleo, fight food lies, and reclaim your health. Victory Belt Publishing, Inc.

Taubes, G. (2018). *The case against Sugar.* Portobello Books.

Taubes, G. (2011). *Why we get fat and what to do about it.* Alfred A. Knopf.

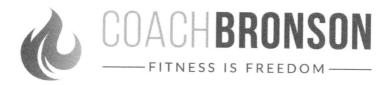

When you're finished reading this book, you will be looking for ways to make some changes and start moving in the right direction. Lucky for you, I've created programs to help you get started!

My F2 Method Programs are the only programs that combine all the concepts from this book and my years of practical, hands-on experience into one solution. No matter where you are, there's a way for you to get started

Find out which program will work best for you! Take the quiz here: https://coachbronson.com/quiz/

References

Boost your immune system

Centers for Disease Control and Prevention. (2020, February 27). *Products - data briefs - number 360 - February 2020.* Centers for Disease Control and Prevention. Retrieved January 23, 2022, from https://www.cdc.gov/nchs/products/databriefs/db360.htm

Centers for Disease Control and Prevention. (2020, August 28). *National Diabetes Statistics Report, 2020.* Centers for Disease Control and Prevention. Retrieved January 23, 2022, from https://www.cdc.gov/diabetes/data/statistics-report/index.html

Explore arthritis in the United States: 2021 annual report. America's Health Rankings. (n.d.). Retrieved January 23, 2022, from https://www.americashealthrankings.org/explore/annual/measure/Arthritis/state/ALL

Explore high blood pressure in the United States: 2021 annual report. America's Health Rankings. (n.d.). Retrieved January 23, 2022, from https://www.americashealthrankings.org/explore/annual/measure/Hypertension/state/ALL

ScienceDaily. (2020, June 15). *Muscles support a strong immune system.* ScienceDaily. Retrieved January 23, 2022, from https://www.sciencedaily.com/releases/2020/06/200615092747.htm

Skeletal muscle as potential central link between sarcopenia and immune senescence. (2019, October 16). Retrieved January 23, 2022, from https://www.thelancet.com/article/S2352-3964(19)30704-2/fulltext

Seyfried, T. N., & Mukherjee, P. (2005, October 21). *Targeting energy metabolism in brain cancer: Review and hypothesis - nutrition & metabolism.* BioMed Central. Retrieved January 23, 2022, from https://nutritionandmetabolism.biomedcentral.com/articles/10.1186/1743-7075-2-30#sec4

You need more muscle

ACSM's guidelines for exercise testing and prescription ... (n.d.). Retrieved January 23, 2022, from https://www.acsm.org/docs/default-source/publications-files/getp10_tables-4-4-4-5-updated.pdf

Frequently asked questions. Frequently Asked Questions | Omron Healthcare. (n.d.). Retrieved January 23, 2022, from https://www.omronhealthcare-ap.com/sg/faqs/weight-management

MediLexicon International. (n.d.). *Body fat percentage chart: Women, men, and calculations.* Medical News Today. Retrieved January 23, 2022, from https://www.medicalnewstoday.com/articles/body-fat-percentage-chart#chart

Gallagher, G., & Heymsfield, S. B. (2000, September 1). *Healthy percentage body fat ranges: an approach for developing guidelines based on body mass index.* Academic.oup.com. Retrieved January 23, 2022, from https://academic.oup.com/ajcn/article/72/3/694/4729363

Surgery, aD. of C. (2018, May). *Study on body composition and its correlation with obesity: ... : Medicine.* LWW. Retrieved January 23, 2022, from https://journals.lww.com/md-journal/Fulltext/2018/05250/Study_on_body_composition_and_its_correlation_with.24.aspx

Macek, P., Biskup, M., Terek-Derszniak, M., Stachura, M., Krol, H., Gozdz, S., & Zak, M. (2020, May 12). *Optimal body fat percentage cut-off values in predicting the obesity-R: DMSO*. Diabetes, Metabolic Syndrome and Obesity: Targets and Therapy. Retrieved January 23, 2022, from https://www.dovepress.com/optimal-body-fat-percentage-cut-off-values-in-predicting-the-obesity-r-peer-reviewed-fulltext-article-DMSO

Kwon, E., Nah, E.-H., Kim, S., & Cho, S. (2021, December 14). *Relative lean body mass and waist circumference for the identification of metabolic syndrome in the Korean general population*. MDPI. Retrieved January 23, 2022, from https://www.mdpi.com/1660-4601/18/24/13186/htm

He, N., Zhang, Y., Zhang, L., Zhang, S., & Ye, H. (2021, December 9). *Relationship between sarcopenia and cardiovascular diseases in the elderly: An overview*. Frontiers in cardiovascular medicine. Retrieved January 23, 2022, from https://www.ncbi.nlm.nih.gov/pmc/articles/PMC8695853/

AS;, S. P. H. A. L. K. (n.d.). Sarcopenia exacerbates obesity-associated insulin resistance and dysglycemia: Findings from the National Health and Nutrition Examination Survey III. PloS one. Retrieved January 23, 2022, from https://pubmed.ncbi.nlm.nih.gov/22421977/

AS;, S. P. K. (n.d.). Relative muscle mass is inversely associated with insulin resistance and prediabetes. findings from the Third National Health and Nutrition Examination Survey. The Journal of clinical endocrinology and metabolism. Retrieved January 23, 2022, from https://pubmed.ncbi.nlm.nih.gov/21778224/

Atlantis E;Martin SA;Haren MT;Taylor AW;Wittert GA; ; (n.d.). *Inverse associations between muscle mass, strength, and the metabolic syndrome*. Metabolism: clinical and experimental. Retrieved January 23, 2022, from https://pubmed.ncbi.nlm.nih.gov/19394973/

Walowski, C. O., Braun, W., Maisch, M. J., Jensen, B., Peine, S., Norman, K., Müller, M. J., & Bosy-Westphal, A. (2020, March 12). *Reference values for skeletal muscle mass – current concepts and methodological considerations.* MDPI. Retrieved February 3, 2022, from https://www.mdpi.com/2072-6643/12/3/755

How to build muscle

Schoenfeld, B. J., & Aragon, A. A. (2018, February 27). How much protein can the body use in a single meal for muscle-building? implications for daily protein distribution - journal of the International Society of Sports Nutrition. BioMed Central. Retrieved March 27, 2022, from https://jissn.biomedcentral.com/articles/10.1186/s12970-018-0215-1

Moore, D. R. (1AD, January 1). Maximizing Post-exercise anabolism: The case for relative protein intakes. Frontiers. Retrieved March 27, 2022, from https://www.frontiersin.org/articles/-10.3389/fnut.2019.00147/full

Hirotsu, C., Tufik, S., & Andersen, M. L. (2015, November). *Interactions between sleep, stress, and metabolism: From physiological to pathological conditions.* Sleep science (Sao Paulo, Brazil). Retrieved January 23, 2022, from https://www.ncbi.nlm.nih.gov/pmc/articles/PMC4688585/

Wittert, G. (2014). *The relationship between sleep disorders and testosterone in men.* Asian journal of andrology. Retrieved January 23, 2022, from https://www.ncbi.nlm.nih.gov/pmc/articles/PMC3955336/

Breushttps://thesleepdoctor.com/author/dr-michael-breus/, D. M. (2021, August 26). *Testosterone, sleep and sexual health.* The Sleep Doctor. Retrieved January 23, 2022, from https://thesleepdoctor.com/2011/10/03/testosterone-sleep-and-sexual-health/

Chennaoui M;Arnal PJ;Drogou C;Sauvet F;Gomez-Merino D; (n.d.). *Sleep extension increases IGF-I concentrations before and during sleep deprivation in healthy young men.* Applied physiology, nutrition, and metabolism = Physiologie appliquee, nutrition et metabolisme. Retrieved January 23, 2022, from https://pubmed.ncbi.nlm.nih.gov/27560704/

Prinz PN;Moe KE;Dulberg EM;Larsen LH;Vitiello MV;Toivola B;Merriam GR; (n.d.). *Higher plasma IGF-1 levels are associated with increased Delta Sleep in healthy older men.* The journals of gerontology. Series A, Biological sciences and medical sciences. Retrieved January 23, 2022, from https://pubmed.ncbi.nlm.nih.gov/7614245/

Velloso, C. P. (2008, June). *Regulation of muscle mass by growth hormone and IGF-I.* British journal of pharmacology. Retrieved January 23, 2022, from https://www.ncbi.nlm.nih.gov/pmc/articles/PMC2439518/

Adams, G. R. (2001, July). *Insulin-like growth factor in muscle growth and its potential abuse by athletes.* Western Journal of Medicine. Retrieved January 23, 2022, from https://www.ncbi.nlm.nih.gov/pmc/articles/PMC1071449/

Takahashi, Y., Kipnis, D. M., & Daughaday, W. H. (1968, September). *Growth hormone secretion during sleep.* The Journal of clinical investigation. Retrieved January 23, 2022, from https://www.ncbi.nlm.nih.gov/pmc/articles/PMC297368/

Tavares, A. B. W., Micmacher, E., Biesek, S., Assumpção, R., Redorat, R., Veloso, U., Vaisman, M., Farinatti, P. T. V., & Conceição, F. (2013). *Effects of growth hormone administration on muscle strength in men over 50 years old.* International journal of endocrinology. Retrieved January 23, 2022, from https://www.ncbi.nlm.nih.gov/pmc/articles/PMC3870652/

How much sleep do you need to build muscle? (9 studies). Sleep And Muscle Growth: How Much Sleep Do You Need? (9 Studies). (n.d.). Retrieved January 23, 2022, from https://builtwithscience.com/sleep-and-muscle-growth/

What to look for in a fitness program

Glassman, G. (2007, April 1). *Understanding CrossFit.* CrossFit Journal. Retrieved January 24, 2022, from http://journal.crossfit.com/2007/04/understanding-crossfit-by-greg.tpl

Glassman, G. (2002, October 21). *What is fitness?* CrossFit. Retrieved January 24, 2022, from https://journal.crossfit.com/article/what-is-fitness

Eating less and still getting fat

Lee, K. (2016, December 6). *Muscle mass and body fat in relation to cardiovascular risk estimation and lipid-lowering eligibility.* Journal of Clinical Densitometry. Retrieved January 23, 2022, from https://www.sciencedirect.com/science/article/abs/pii/S1094 695016302529

E;, L. P. D. B. A. H. J. S. (n.d.). *Healthy lifestyle characteristics and their joint association with cardiovascular disease biomarkers in US adults.* Mayo Clinic proceedings. Retrieved January 23, 2022, from https://pubmed.ncbi.nlm.nih.gov/26906650/

Rivero, E. (2016, April 18). *Higher muscle mass associated with lower mortality risk in people with heart disease.* UCLA. Retrieved January 23, 2022, from https://newsroom.ucla.edu/releases/higher-muscle-mass-associated-with-lower-mortality-risk-in-people-with-heart-disease

Saito, Y., Takahashi, O., Arioka, H., & Kobayashi, D. (2017, April 3). *Associations between body fat variability and later onset of cardiovascular disease risk factors*. PloS one. Retrieved January 23, 2022, from https://www.ncbi.nlm.nih.gov/pmc/articles/PMC5378370/

How to fight diabetes with improved body composition. InBody USA. (2020, January 13). Retrieved January 23, 2022, from https://inbodyusa.com/blogs/inbodyblog/how-to-fight-diabetes-with-improved-body-composition/

Zeng, Q., Dong, S.-Y., Sun, X.-N., Xie, J., & Cui, Y. (2012, July). *Percent body fat is a better predictor of cardiovascular risk factors than body mass index*. Brazilian journal of medical and biological research = Revista brasileira de pesquisas medicas e biologicas. Retrieved January 23, 2022, from https://www.ncbi.nlm.nih.gov/pmc/articles/PMC3854278/

Eating more and getting skinny

Walton, C. M., Jacobsen, S. M., Dallon, B. W., Saito, E. R., Bennett, S. L. H., Davidson, L. E., Thomson, D. M., Hyldahl, R. D., & Bikman, B. T. (2020, August 29). *Ketones elicit distinct alterations in adipose mitochondrial bioenergetics*. MDPI. Retrieved January 23, 2022, from https://www.mdpi.com/1422-0067/21/17/6255

Pesta, D., I, D. of D. R., Hoppel, F., Science, D. of S., Macek, C., Messner, H., Faulhaber, M., Kobel, C., Statistics, D. of M., Parson, W., Medicine, I. of L., Burtscher, M., Schocke, M., Gnaiger, E., Laboratory, D. S. R., PJ, A., L, B., VS, B., AD, B., … Jacobs, R. A. (2011, October 1). *Similar qualitative and quantitative changes of mitochondrial respiration following strength and endurance training in normoxia and hypoxia in sedentary humans*. American Journal of Physiology-Regulatory, Integrative and Comparative Physiology. Retrieved January 23, 2022, from https://journals.physiology.org/doi/full/10.1152/ajpregu.00285.2011

Wang L;Mascher H;Psilander N;Blomstrand E;Sahlin K; (n.d.). Resistance exercise enhances the molecular signaling of mitochondrial biogenesis induced by endurance exercise in human skeletal muscle. Journal of applied physiology (Bethesda, Md. : 1985). Retrieved January 23, 2022, from https://pubmed.ncbi.nlm.nih.gov/21836044/

Managing your mitochondria. Mark's Daily Apple. (2013, October 25). Retrieved January 23, 2022, from https://www.marksdailyapple.com/managing-your-mitochondria/

Seyfried, T. N., & Mukherjee, P. (2005, October 21). *Targeting energy metabolism in brain cancer: Review and hypothesis - nutrition & metabolism.* BioMed Central. Retrieved January 23, 2022, from https://nutritionandmetabolism.biomedcentral.com/articles/10.1186/1743-7075-2-30#sec4

Srivastava, S., Baxa, U., Niu, G., Chen, X., & Veech, R. L. (2013, January). *A ketogenic diet increases brown adipose tissue mitochondrial proteins and UCP1 levels in mice.* IUBMB life. Retrieved January 23, 2022, from https://www.ncbi.nlm.nih.gov/pmc/articles/PMC3821007/

Li, X., Higashida, K., Kawamura, T., & Higuchi, M. (2016, April 6). *Alternate-day high-fat diet induces an increase in mitochondrial enzyme activities and protein content in rat skeletal muscle.* Nutrients. Retrieved January 23, 2022, from https://www.ncbi.nlm.nih.gov/pmc/articles/PMC4848672/

Keto and alcohol don't mix

Cederbaum, A. I. (2012, November). *Alcohol metabolism.* Clinics in liver disease. Retrieved January 23, 2022, from https://www.ncbi.nlm.nih.gov/pmc/articles/PMC3484320/

Guo, R., & Ren, J. (2010, April). *Alcohol and acetaldehyde in Public Health: From Marvel to menace.* International journal of environmental research and public health. Retrieved January 23, 2022, from https://www.ncbi.nlm.nih.gov/pmc/articles/PMC2872347/

U.S. Department of Health and Human Services. (n.d.). *Alcohol alert.* National Institute on Alcohol Abuse and Alcoholism. Retrieved January 23, 2022, from https://pubs.niaaa.nih.gov/publications/arh25-2/101-109.htm

Choose your carbs wisely

Encyclopædia Britannica, inc. (n.d.). *Cellulose.* Encyclopædia Britannica. Retrieved January 23, 2022, from https://www.britannica.com/science/cellulose

Kamba, A., Daimon, M., Murakami, H., Otaka, H., Matsuki, K., Sato, E., Tanabe, J., Takayasu, S., Matsuhashi, Y., Yanagimachi, M., Terui, K., Kageyama, K., Tokuda, I., Takahashi, I., & Nakaji, S. (2016, November 18). *Association between higher serum cortisol levels and decreased insulin secretion in a general population.* PloS one. Retrieved January 23, 2022, from https://www.ncbi.nlm.nih.gov/pmc/articles/PMC5115704/

Straub, R. H. (2014, February 13). *Interaction of the endocrine system with inflammation: A function of energy and volume regulation.* Arthritis research & therapy. Retrieved January 23, 2022, from https://www.ncbi.nlm.nih.gov/pmc/articles/PMC3978663/

Garcia-Leme, J., & Farsky, S. P. (1993). *Hormonal control of inflammatory responses.* Mediators of inflammation. Retrieved January 23, 2022, from https://www.ncbi.nlm.nih.gov/pmc/articles/PMC2365405/

Petroski, W., & Minich, D. M. (2020, September 24). *Is there such a thing as "anti-nutrients"? A narrative review of perceived problematic plant compounds*. Nutrients. Retrieved January 23, 2022, from https://www.ncbi.nlm.nih.gov/pmc/articles/PMC7600777/

Levy, J. (2020, June 10). *10 antinutrients to get out of your diet immediately*. Dr. Axe. Retrieved January 23, 2022, from https://draxe.com/nutrition/antinutrients/

Antinutrients. Antinutrients - an overview | ScienceDirect Topics. (n.d.). Retrieved January 23, 2022, from https://www.sciencedirect.com/topics/food-science/-antinutrients

Samtiya, M., Aluko, R. E., & Dhewa, T. (2020, March 6). *Plant food anti-nutritional factors and their reduction strategies: An Overview - food production, processing and Nutrition*. BioMed Central. Retrieved January 23, 2022, from https://fppn.biomedcentral.com/articles/10.1186/s43014-020-0020-5

Vitamins and minerals on a ketogenic diet

Listing of vitamins. Harvard Health. (2020, August 31). Retrieved January 23, 2022, from https://www.health.harvard.edu/staying-healthy/listing_of_vitamins

Nutrition Data and Food Facts. Nutrition Data know what you eat. (n.d.). Retrieved January 23, 2022, from https://nutritiondata.self.com/

Emmerich, M., & Emmerich, C. (2018). Nutrients in Superfoods Compared to Animal Protein. In *Keto. The Complete Guide to success on the ketogenic diet, including simplified science and no-cook meal plans*. essay, Victory Belt Publishing Inc.

More about protein

Antonio J;Ellerbroek A;Silver T;Vargas L;Tamayo A;Buehn R;Peacock CA; (n.d.). *A high protein diet has no harmful effects: A one-year crossover study in resistance-trained males.* Journal of nutrition and metabolism. Retrieved January 23, 2022, from https://pubmed.ncbi.nlm.nih.gov/27807480/

Antonio J;Ellerbroek A;Silver T;Vargas L;Peacock C; (n.d.). *The effects of a high protein Diet on indices of health and body composition--a crossover trial in resistance-trained men.* Journal of the International Society of Sports Nutrition. Retrieved January 23, 2022, from https://pubmed.ncbi.nlm.nih.gov/26778925/

Campbell BI;Aguilar D;Conlin L;Vargas A;Schoenfeld BJ;Corson A;Gai C;Best S;Galvan E;Couvillion K; (n.d.). Effects of high versus low protein intake on body composition and maximal strength in aspiring female physique athletes engaging in an 8-week resistance training program. International journal of sport nutrition and exercise metabolism. Retrieved January 23, 2022, from https://pubmed.ncbi.nlm.nih.gov/29405780/

Learn the facts: Does excess dietary protein get stored as fat? written by Dylan Klein. SimplyShredded.com | The Ultimate Lifting Experience. (2014, March 26). Retrieved January 23, 2022, from http://simplyshredded.com/does-excess-protein-get-stored-as-fat.html

Steffanson Bellvue Experiment - borntoeatmeat.com. PROLONGED MEAT DIETS WITH A STUDY OF KIDNEY FUNCTION AND KETOSIS. (1930). Retrieved January 23, 2022, from https://borntoeatmeat.com/wp-content/uploads/2017/10/-Steffanson-Bellvue-Experiment.pdf, p. 666-667

Gluconeogenesis supports a ketogenic diet

L;, L. (n.d.). *Ketone bodies: A review of Physiology, Pathophysiology and application of monitoring to diabetes.* Diabetes/metabolism research and reviews. Retrieved January 31, 2022, from https://pubmed.ncbi.nlm.nih.gov/10634967/

Melkonian, E. A. (2021, May 9). *Physiology, gluconeogenesis.* StatPearls [Internet]. Retrieved January 31, 2022, from https://www.ncbi.nlm.nih.gov/books/NBK541119/

Dhillon, K. K. (2021, February 17). *Biochemistry, ketogenesis.* StatPearls [Internet]. Retrieved January 31, 2022, from https://www.ncbi.nlm.nih.gov/books/NBK493179/

You Can Get There From Here: Acetone, Anionic Ketones and Even-Carbon Fatty Acids can Provide Substrates for Gluconeogenesis. Ketogenesis explained. (n.d.). Retrieved January 31, 2022, from https://everything.explained.today/Ketogenesis/

Ketogenesis. Ketogenesis - an overview | ScienceDirect Topics. (n.d.). Retrieved January 31, 2022, from https://www.sciencedirect.com/topics/medicine-and-dentistry/ketogenesis

Libretexts. (2021, January 3). *5.3b: Pyruvic acid and metabolism.* Biology LibreTexts. Retrieved January 31, 2022, from https://bio.libretexts.org/Bookshelves/Microbiology/Book%3A_Microbiology_(Boundless)/5%3A_Microbial_Metabolism/5.03%3A_Catabolism/5.3B%3A_Pyruvic_Acid_and_Metabolism

MS;, P. T. B. B. L. L. O. (n.d.). *The stimulation of hepatic gluconeogenesis by acetoacetate precursors. A role for the monocarboxylate translocator.* The Journal of biological chemistry. Retrieved January 31, 2022, from https://pubmed.ncbi.nlm.nih.gov/6736017/

Hui, S., Ghergurovich, J. M., Morscher, R. J., Jang, C., Teng, X., Lu, W., Esparza, L. A., Reya, T., Le Zhan, Yanxiang Guo, J., White, E., & Rabinowitz, J. D. (2017, November 2). *Glucose feeds the TCA cycle via circulating lactate.* Nature. Retrieved January 31, 2022, from https://www.ncbi.nlm.nih.gov/pmc/articles/PMC5898814/

Acetoacetate: What is it, why it's important & the Benefits. Ruled Me. (2022, January 31). Retrieved January 31, 2022, from https://www.ruled.me/what-is-acetoacetate/

London : Biochemical Society. (1987, January 1). *Krebs' citric acid cycle: Half a century and still turning.* Internet Archive. Retrieved January 31, 2022, from https://archive.org/details/krebscitricacidc0000unse/page/25/mode/2up

Events. Events | Institute for Translational Medicine and Therapeutics | Perelman School of Medicine at the University of Pennsylvania. (n.d.). Retrieved January 31, 2022, from https://www.med.upenn.edu/itmat/events/

Wikimedia Foundation. (2022, January 31). *Cori cycle.* Wikipedia. Retrieved January 31, 2022, from https://en.wikipedia.org/wiki/Cori_cycle

Wikimedia Foundation. (2022, January 26). *Citric acid cycle.* Wikipedia. Retrieved January 31, 2022, from https://en.wikipedia.org/wiki/Citric_acid_cycle#Glucose_feeds_the_TCA_cycle_via_circulating_lactate

Wikimedia Foundation. (2022, January 18). *Ketogenesis.* Wikipedia. Retrieved January 31, 2022, from https://en.wikipedia.org/wiki/Ketogenesis

The cholesterol myth

MD, P. M., 29, P. M. M. D. on J., 30, P. M. M. D. on J., & *, N. (n.d.). *I went zero carb and my total and LDL cholesterol went really high! is that dangerous? no!* Zero Carb Doc. Retrieved January 26, 2022, from http://borntoeatmeat.com/i-went-zero-carb-and-my-total-and-ldl-cholesterol-went-really-high-is-that-dangerous-no/

Malhotra, A. (2013, October 22). *Saturated fat is not the major issue.* The BMJ. Retrieved January 26, 2022, from https://www.bmj.com/content/347/bmj.f6340.full

Ramsden CE;Zamora D;Majchrzak-Hong S;Faurot KR;Broste SK;Frantz RP;Davis JM;Ringel A;Suchindran CM;Hibbeln JR; (n.d.). *Re-evaluation of the traditional diet-heart hypothesis: Analysis of recovered data from Minnesota Coronary Experiment (1968-73).* BMJ (Clinical research ed.). Retrieved January 26, 2022, from https://pubmed.ncbi.nlm.nih.gov/27071971/

Ravnskov, U., Diamond, D. M., Hama, R., Hamazaki, T., Hammarskjöld, B., Hynes, N., Kendrick, M., Langsjoen, P. H., Malhotra, A., Mascitelli, L., McCully, K. S., Ogushi, Y., Okuyama, H., Rosch, P. J., Schersten, T., Sultan, S., & Sundberg, R. (2016, June 1). *Lack of an association or an inverse association between low-density-lipoprotein cholesterol and mortality in the elderly: A systematic review.* BMJ Open. Retrieved January 26, 2022, from https://bmjopen.bmj.com/content/6/6/e010401

Forsythe CE;Phinney SD;Feinman RD;Volk BM;Freidenreich D;Quann E;Ballard K;Puglisi MJ;Maresh CM;Kraemer WJ;Bibus DM;Fernandez ML;Volek JS; (n.d.). *Limited effect of dietary saturated fat on plasma saturated fat in the context of a low carbohydrate diet.* Lipids. Retrieved January 26, 2022, from https://pubmed.ncbi.nlm.nih.gov/20820932/

Harcombe, Z., Baker, J. S., Cooper, S. M., Davies, B., Sculthorpe, N., DiNicolantonio, J. J., & Grace, F. (2015, January 1). Evidence from randomised controlled trials did not support the introduction of dietary fat guidelines in 1977 and 1983: A systematic review and meta-analysis. Open Heart. Retrieved January 26, 2022, from https://openheart.bmj.com/content/2/1/e000196

Sung KC;Huh JH;Ryu S;Lee JY;Scorletti E;Byrne CD;Kim JY;Hyun DS;Ko SB; (n.d.). *Low levels of low-density lipoprotein cholesterol and mortality outcomes in non-statin users.* Journal of clinical medicine. Retrieved January 26, 2022, from https://pubmed.ncbi.nlm.nih.gov/31581520/

Lee, J. H., Duster, M., Roberts, T., & Devinsky, O. (1AD, January 1). United States dietary trends since 1800: Lack of association between saturated fatty acid consumption and non-communicable diseases. Frontiers. Retrieved January 26, 2022, from https://www.frontiersin.org/articles/10.3389/fnut.2021.748847/full

Krans, B. (2016, June 25). *LDL cholesterol: 'bad' cholesterol may not be so bad.* Healthline. Retrieved January 26, 2022, from https://www.healthline.com/health-news/bad-cholesterol-may-have-bad-rap

Watermark-Silverchair-com.ezproxy1.library.arizona.edu. Ratio of Triglycerides to HDL Cholesterol Is an Indicator of LDL Particle Size in Patients With Type 2 Diabetes and Normal HDL Cholesterol Levels. (n.d.). Retrieved January 26, 2022, from https://watermark-silverchair-com.ezproxy1.library.arizona.edu/bltn08102.pdf

The Definitive Guide to Cholesterol. Mark's Daily Apple. (2020, June 26). Retrieved January 26, 2022, from https://www.marksdailyapple.com/cholesterol/

Rosamond, W. G. M. W., Members, W. G., Search for more papers by this author, Rosamond, W., Wayne Rosamond Search for more papers by this author, Flegal, K., Katherine Flegal Search for more papers by this author, Furie, K., Karen Furie Search for more papers by this author, Go, A., Alan Go Search for more papers by this author, Greenlund, K., Kurt Greenlund Search for more papers by this author, Haase, N., Nancy Haase Search for more papers by this author, Hailpern, S. M., Susan M. Hailpern Search for more papers by this author, Ho, M., Michael Ho Search for more papers by this author, … Yuling Hong Search for more papers by this author. (2007, December 17). *Heart disease and stroke statistics-2008 update.* Circulation. Retrieved January 31, 2022, from https://www.ahajournals.org/doi/full/10.1161/CIRCUL ATIONAHA.107.187998

Lee, J. H., Duster, M., Roberts, T., & Devinsky, O. (1AD, January 1). United States dietary trends since 1800: Lack of association between saturated fatty acid consumption and non-communicable diseases. Frontiers. Retrieved January 31, 2022, from https://www.frontiersin.org/articles/10.3389/fnut.2021.74884 7/full

Knobbe, C. A., & Stojanoska, M. (2017, October 14). The 'displacing foods of modern commerce' are the primary and proximate cause of age-related macular degeneration: A unifying singular hypothesis. Medical Hypotheses. Retrieved January 31, 2022, from https://www.sciencedirect.com/science/article/pii/S03069877 17305017#f0010

Children & Cardiovascular Diseases - heart.org. (n.d.). Retrieved January 31, 2022, from https://www.heart.org/idc/groups/heart-public/@wcm/@sop/@smd/documents/downloadable/ucm _483966.pdf

Ferreira-González, I. (2014, February 1). *The epidemiology of coronary heart disease: Revista Española de Cardiología.* Revista Española de Cardiología (English Edition). Retrieved January 31, 2022, from https://www.revespcardiol.org/en-the-epidemiology-coronary-heart-disease-articulo-S1885585713003381

Ng CY;Leong XF;Masbah N;Adam SK;Kamisah Y;Jaarin K; (n.d.). *Heated vegetable oils and cardiovascular disease risk factors.* Vascular pharmacology. Retrieved January 31, 2022, from https://pubmed.ncbi.nlm.nih.gov/24632108/

DiNicolantonio, J. J., & O'Keefe, J. H. (2018, September 26). *Omega-6 vegetable oils as a driver of coronary heart disease: The oxidized linoleic acid hypothesis.* Open heart. Retrieved January 31, 2022, from https://www.ncbi.nlm.nih.gov/pmc/articles/PMC6196963/#:~:text=In%20summary%2C%20numerous%20lines%20of,of%20industrial%20seed%20oils%20commonly

Kresser, C. (2019, September 23). *How industrial seed oils are making us sick.* How Industrial Seed Oils Are Making Us Sick. Retrieved January 31, 2022, from https://chriskresser.com/how-industrial-seed-oils-are-making-us-sick/

Salt is not the problem

Centers for Disease Control and Prevention. (2021, September 27). *Facts about hypertension.* Centers for Disease Control and Prevention. Retrieved February 9, 2022, from https://www.cdc.gov/bloodpressure/facts.htm

Chen L;Caballero B;Mitchell DC;Loria C;Lin PH;Champagne CM;Elmer PJ;Ard JD;Batch BC;Anderson CA;Appel LJ; (n.d.). Reducing consumption of sugar-sweetened beverages is associated with reduced blood pressure: A prospective study among United States Adults. Circulation. Retrieved February 9, 2022, from https://pubmed.ncbi.nlm.nih.gov/20497980/

Cordain L;Eaton SB;Sebastian A;Mann N;Lindeberg S;Watkins BA;O'Keefe JH;Brand-Miller J; (n.d.). *Origins and evolution of the Western Diet: Health Implications for the 21st Century.* The American journal of clinical nutrition. Retrieved February 9, 2022, from https://pubmed.ncbi.nlm.nih.gov/15699220/

M;, H. (n.d.). *The role of magnesium in hypertension and cardiovascular disease.* Journal of clinical hypertension (Greenwich, Conn.). Retrieved February 9, 2022, from https://pubmed.ncbi.nlm.nih.gov/22051430/

A;, R. (n.d.). *[magnesium and hypertension].* Clinical calcium. Retrieved February 9, 2022, from https://pubmed.ncbi.nlm.nih.gov/15692166/

Zhang, X., Xi Zhang From the Department of Epidemiology, Li, Y., Yufeng Li From the Department of Epidemiology, Gobbo, L. C. D., Liana C. Del Gobbo From the Department of Epidemiology, Rosanoff, A., Andrea Rosanoff From the Department of Epidemiology, Wang, J., Jiawei Wang From the Department of Epidemiology, Zhang, W., Wen Zhang From the Department of Epidemiology, Song, Y., Yiqing Song From the Department of Epidemiology, & *These authors contributed equally to this work.The online-only Data Supplement is available with this article at http://hyper.ahajournals.org/lookup/suppl/doi:10.1161/HYPERTENSIONAHA.116.07664/-/DC1.Correspondence to Yiqing Song. (2016, July 11). *Effects of magnesium supplementation on blood pressure.* Hypertension. Retrieved February 9, 2022, from https://www.ahajournals.org/doi/10.1161/hypertensionaha.116.07664

Key minerals to help control blood pressure. Harvard Health. (2019, May 3). Retrieved February 9, 2022, from https://www.health.harvard.edu/heart-health/key-minerals-to-help-control-blood-pressure

A primal guide to blood pressure: 8 common (and not so common) interventions. Mark's Daily Apple. (2019, October 16). Retrieved February 9, 2022, from https://www.marksdailyapple.com/8-blood-pressure-interventions/

O'Donnell MJ;Yusuf S;Mente A;Gao P;Mann JF;Teo K;McQueen M;Sleight P;Sharma AM;Dans A;Probstfield J;Schmieder RE; (n.d.). *Urinary sodium and potassium excretion and risk of cardiovascular events.* JAMA. Retrieved February 9, 2022, from https://pubmed.ncbi.nlm.nih.gov/22110105/

From the desk of Robb Wolf, & Wolf, R. (n.d.). *Electrolytes and heart health: A science-based guide.* Drink LMNT, INC. Retrieved February 9, 2022, from https://drinklmnt.com/blogs/health/electrolytes-and-heart-health

says:, A. D., says:, H. M., says:, S. G., says:, J. B., says:, M., Says:, R., says:, S., says:, A., says:, D., Says:, S. A., says:, S. H. E. I. L. A., Says:, M., says:, S., says:, D. J. P., says:, P. S., says:, S. R., says:, A. dixit, Says:, S., says:, katherine M., … says:, M. (2014, June 20). *How (and why) to lower your blood pressure naturally.* Chris Kresser. Retrieved February 9, 2022, from https://chriskresser.com/how-and-why-to-lower-your-blood-pressure-naturally/

Salvetti A;Brogi G;Di Legge V;Bernini GP; (n.d.). *The inter-relationship between insulin resistance and hypertension.* Drugs. Retrieved February 9, 2022, from https://pubmed.ncbi.nlm.nih.gov/7512468

Zhou, M.-S., Wang, A., & Yu, H. (2014, January 31). *Link between insulin resistance and hypertension: What is the evidence from evolutionary biology?* Diabetology & metabolic syndrome. Retrieved February 9, 2022, from https://www.ncbi.nlm.nih.gov/pmc/articles/PMC3996172/

Low-salt diet increases insulin resistance in healthy subjects. (n.d.). Retrieved February 9, 2022, from https://www.metabolismjournal.com/article/S0026-0495(10)00329-X/fulltext

Ekinci, E. I., Clarke, S., Thomas, M. C., Moran, J. L., Cheong, K., MacIsaac, R. J., & Jerums, G. (2011, February 17). *Dietary salt intake and mortality in patients with type 2 diabetes.* American Diabetes Association. Retrieved February 9, 2022, from https://diabetesjournals.org/care/article/34/3/703/38793/Dietary-Salt-Intake-and-Mortality-in-Patients-With

Katarzyna Stolarz-Skrzypek, M. D. (2011, May 4). *Fatal and nonfatal outcomes, incidence of hypertension, and blood pressure changes in relation to urinary sodium excretion.* JAMA. Retrieved February 9, 2022, from https://jamanetwork.com/journals/jama/fullarticle/899663

Flicker L;Almeida OP;Acres J;Le MT;Tuohy RJ;Jamrozik K;Hankey G;Norman P; (n.d.). *Predictors of impaired cognitive function in men over the age of 80 years: Results from the Health in Men Study.* Age and ageing. Retrieved February 9, 2022, from https://pubmed.ncbi.nlm.nih.gov/15591486/

Renneboog B;Musch W;Vandemergel X;Manto MU;Decaux G; (n.d.). *Mild chronic hyponatremia is associated with falls, unsteadiness, and attention deficits.* The American journal of medicine. Retrieved February 9, 2022, from https://pubmed.ncbi.nlm.nih.gov/16431193/

Satin, M., Lipson, C., Claydon, J., Anna, Kunkle, R., Hyrum, Gwen, Samantha, Thomson, G., Boyd, T., Henry, Brooks, Ahmed, S., John, D. U., Chris, Bob, Colbin, A., Hogel, L., Hogel, L., … speedstarr35. (2020, October 4). *Salt and our health.* The Weston A. Price Foundation. Retrieved February 9, 2022, from https://www.westonaprice.org/health-topics/abcs-of-nutrition/salt-and-our-health/